Julia Maitret

# VEGETARIAN MENUS

## And everything you need to know about nutrition

authorHOUSE®

*AuthorHouse™*
*1663 Liberty Drive, Suite 200*
*Bloomington, IN 47403*
*www.authorhouse.com*
*Phone: 1-800-839-8640*

*First published by AuthorHouse    3/26/2009*

*ISBN: 978-1-4343-6257-5 (sc)*

*Printed in the United States of America*
*Bloomington, Indiana*

*This book is printed on acid-free paper.*

Dedicated to:
- My Inner Guide, with my heartfelt love.
- The memory of my beloved parents: Julio and María.
- My beloved daughters: Elianne and Andrea, my treasures.
- The memory of my beloved son and daughter: Eduardo and Jeannine
- My beloved grandchildren: Daniella and Patricio.
- My dearest sisters: Fonsi and Amada, and their families
- The memory of my sisters Emilia, Blanca, and Regina, and to their families.
- The memory of my brother Julio and his family
- The people of San Rafael Veracruz, Mexico birthplace of my beloved father.
- And to all those who promote animal rights.
- And to all those who promote ecological conscience.

# Acknowledgements

I wish to thank with all my heart all those wonderful people who directly or indirectly stimulated my interest in vegetarianism some thirty-three years ago and who still do so.

To my dear friend Salvador Flores (Abdala) who passed me the telephone and gave me the telephone number of the naturist doctor. In particular, I would like to thank Carlos Michan Amiga, architect, naturist doctor and maestro, who with boundless friendship, patience and knowledge helped me to recover from serious illness and this discipline guided my life towards my inner conscience. To Harish Johari, whose teachings of Indian cuisine directly contributed to all that I have learned about it.

Thanks to the people who have written books filled with wisdom that have been my major source of learning through this years of vegetarian life-style; which improved my quality of life.

I'd like to thank my daughters Elianne and Andrea for their love and support they've given me in many different ways; and for choosing me as their mother before their birth in this beautiful Planet. Blessings to their souls from my Highest Being.

Special thanks to my daughter Elianne for revising the translation of this book to the English language and that her love and understanding has supported me to overcome the obstacles I've encountered in my path. My love and blessings be with her from my Highest Being.

To Roberto, the father of my daughters, for his invaluable support during the first stage…To my family for its support…To all my friends who understood and respected this change in me, particularly Franca Romani who also went down the road of vegetarianism; to the Vergara Mercado family; to all my close friends and acquaintances whose tasty meat-free recipes have helped me to live contentedly with a vegetarian diet: Myrna Gomez, Gloria Bassaure, Abdala, Gaby Limon, Ruth Shapiro, Jorge Cadiz, Miriam Rojas, Brisia Gorey, Eli, Azari Cuenca, Blanca Chuzeville, Olga Rovirosa, Eva Arana, and many others who escape me for the time being and to whom I apologize for only having included their recipe.

Thanks you to all the loving human beings who helped me in several ways, they are in my heart.

To all my colleagues at the AMA ecology group in Cancun, Quintana Roo, particularly Ligia Medrano to whom I passed on my recipes, who encouraged me to give vegetarian cooking classes. That gave me the idea of putting together this recipe book, and all that I learned through my life.

To Lucero Chavarria, my dear friend, who arrived at the last moment and showed me how to put this book together…THANK YOU ALL.

# Introduction

"The spirit is the life, the mind is the builder, and the body is the outcome"

Edgar Cayce.

Health is a dynamic process of all human body's system in coordinated activity of assimilation and elimination. In this process, the circulatory and nervous systems are vital to achieve a state of balance. Health and well-being depends on ourselves paying attention to the body, the mind, the spirit, and the meditation.

The wisdom of nature focuses on the organism's health that constantly searches for a state of balance.

Some people don't know what to do to feel better or to recover their health, nor do they conceive the idea that they have the ability to improve their health.

Our immune system is made up of cells in charged of fighting, deactivating, and eliminating every intruder that can harm our body.

When working efficiently, the immune system multiplies the possibility of maintaining good health. The immune-deficiency is caused by poor nutrition, consumption of saturated fats, lots of sugars, processed food, and food lacking essentials nutrients, chronic stress, and addictions such as drugs, alcohol, tobacco, and medicines.

Our quality of life depends, mainly, on our health and defenses. It is on achievement to live according to a vegetarian hygiene.

It is right to say that we can't always control certain circumstances and prevent all illnesses because most of them are a product of neglecting our body's needs throughout our lives. Health could be recovered with a proper attitude and an adequate nutrition; curative herbs, and some practices associated with life styles could achieve excellent results that are vital to good health.

Having a goal in life with positive thoughts and feelings and keeping the immune and endocrine systems in optimal conditions will keep us balanced and with energy.

This can be accomplished through a vegetarian life style, gratitude to life, and compassion for every living organism.

It cannot be denied that every action is preceded by a thought and that thoughts "good or bad" are the result of the food we eat.

Krishna said: "Moral conduct, good habits, spiritual effort, all depend upon the quality of the food; diseases, mental weakness, spiritual slackness, all are produced by the wrong foods. Food plays a crucial role in determining one's thoughts, feelings, words and actions".

Some people say that plants are alive too. But plants, fruits and vegetables have no blood, flesh or bones and their conscience level is the lowest and it is not considered violence.

Compassion and non-violence towards all living things are important factors, to be observed by spiritual people and this is accomplished only through a vegetarian life style.

R.N. Lakhotia says: "The truly spiritual people should never think on nourishing their bodies with non-vegetarian food or any other food obtained through cruelty".

Vegetarian food is the only ideal food for mankind from the point of view of health, nutrition, help the starving people, protect the environment, preserve natural resources; as proven scientifically and in accordance with wise men teachings and the words of people who have experienced it and they are inviting us to be compassionate towards animals and to search for and preserve peace.

Paracelsus said: "In each garden plants flourish, they're needed by the inhabitants of each household to have harmony and to be healed."

Let the ecological conscience unite us; and peace and happiness reign in all Beings on Earth.

Julia Maitret

# A Glance At Nutrition

## ENJOYING A BETTER QUALITY OF LIFE

How many times have we asked ourselves if what we eat is suitable for keeping our body healthy, or if we should change our eating habits in order to enjoy better health and to be better nourished?

<u>Nutrients</u> are the substance that cells receive and <u>food</u> is what we eat.

It is scientifically proven that our quality of life is directly related to good eating habits, namely, the quality and quantity of what we should eat. Of the thousands of substances involved in human metabolism, only a few are essential and need to be provided by food, as most substances are produced by the metabolic processes that take place within our organism. So once again, nature shows what it can do to preserve a species. Surely we should ask ourselves: "What is the right food for keeping healthy or improving our health?"

## THE 5 LAWS OF GOOD NUTRITION:

1.  Your diet must be complete and balanced, in other words, it should contain all substances that are indispensable for the proper functioning of our organism, these being: proteins, carbohydrates or sugars, fats or lipids, minerals, vitamins, and water.

2.  Food should be adjusted to the needs or requirements of each individual, depending on age, sex, stature, ideal weight, physical constitution, physical activity and certain special situations: such as pregnancy, breast feeding, childhood, adolescence and periods of convalescence, during which requirements are greater.

3.  You must eat sufficient food, in other words, the amount of food you need to satisfy your appetite, but without going to extremes.

4.  Food must be biologically pure, free of any contaminating organisms and be as natural as possible. The best form of nutrition is that based on natural products. It has been proven that food does its job best, the least it is processed. Nature is never wrong.

5.  Food must be properly prepared and must be pleasant to our senses of sight, smell, and taste.

# FACTORS TO BE TAKEN INTO ACCOUNT FOR NUTRITION

1. **Energy value**. Food should be consumed as fuel for our bodily activities. Carbohydrates are an excellent source of energy and build up reserves. In the form of glucose (sugar) they provide the brain energy (fruit contains fructose which is converted to glucose in the brain). The thyroid gland, in the throat, controls the metabolism of the entire body and needs energy to carry out its functions properly.

2. **Quality of food**. Optimum nutrition is based on eating natural products such as fresh vegetables and fresh and raw seasonal fruits that contain their maximum biological value, thus increasing reserves of enzymes in the digestive system. **What the season produces = Syntony = Balance.** Edgar Cayce, suggests that we should eat food that contains minerals or vibrations of the place where we live, because the body needs them. Lower-quality food increases our desire to eat more, so as to replace the needs of what should be correct nutrition. Eating natural food improves digestion and helps us to get over certain bad eating habits developed by eating overcooked and over processed food, or food with additives.

3. **Amount of food.** The amount of food should be proportional to the needs of each individual, according to age, sex, stature, ideal weight, constitution and physical activity and certain special situations, such as pregnancy, breast feeding, childhood, adolescence and convalescence. Food should be eaten in the right physiological proportion, which should be moderate, as this helps to increase vitality and improve health. Eating too much compresses the digestive system and eating too little stimulates the digestive function: "quantity destroys quality". Eat what you fancy, without exaggerating, and do not eat what you think is too much.

4. **Variety of food.** Food should be prepared properly and be pleasant to the senses of sight, smell and taste. A physiologically balanced diet maintains a balance between what we eat every day. Eat fresh fruit and vegetables, cereals, roots, oleaginous products, leguminous products and juices.

5. **Digestion.** It is recommendable to eat at the same meal food, sustenance that takes the same time to be digested (see Incompatibilities). Food is digested in the stomach at a normal temperature of 37 degrees that increases by drinking cold drinks, eating hot or spicy food, overcooked or devitalized food (cans) and eating too much. This congests mucus, ferments food (the less fermentation, the better your health) and leads to dyspepsia and ulcers. In order to improve digestion, it is recommendable not to eat anything within three hours of having eaten. **Food is more digestible** when you eat naturally, maturely, and at a normal temperature: fruits, vegetables, and whole grains cereals. Eat with appetite and chew solid food well. **Food is more indigestible** at a very advanced stage of maturity, refined cereals, mustard, chili and pepper. Do not take on liquid while eating (because they dilute the gastric juices), do not eat quickly, do not eat if you are not hungry, chew well, and do not get upset while you are eating.

6. **Preparing food.** Food should be prepared simply and hygienically, with very few condiments. Vegetables should be lightly steamed to please the senses.

7. **Cost and economy**. There are some very economical and nutritional products, such as soy beans. They are very cheap and have a high content of proteins and nutrients, as well as being versatile. They also contain properties that help to prevent illness.

8. **The psychological factor**: Albert Einstein, the famous physician and Nobel Prize winner said: "I believe that the vegetarian way of life will have a highly beneficial influence on the destiny of the human race, due to the purely physical effect on human temperament".

9. **Biological function**: bodily activities, development, real nutrients.

10. **A pleasurable function**: eating and drinking properly and with satisfaction.

11. **A social function**: the economy, culture and history.

# GENERAL HYGIENE

**Functions of the organism**: breathing, real nutrients, forming substances and structures, excreting waste, hygiene, physical activity, dreaming, thinking, feeling, etc.

## What is hygiene?

Hygiene consists of healthy, proper and individual eating, with the right combination of food, the right consumption of fruit, vegetables, etc, drinking organic liquids (natural juices), exercising, cleaning the body, fasting and meditating.

## What is sustenance?

A substance is that enters the organism and releases energy to keep it alive.

**Sustenance may include:**

**Plastic:** the solid sustenance that we take on.

**Air:** the air that we breathe through the nose and skin.

**Ethereal:** solar sustenance that provides us heat and energy (called luminous) and that provides us calcium, iron, phosphorous and sulfur.

**Electrical and magnetic:** the balance between these two poles provides the metabolic function that, in turn, gives us health. Apply any of these two quick methods to recover your electrical and magnetic energy:

1. Stand on grass, earth or sand barefoot; open your legs slightly and raise your arms with your palms facing upwards. It is better to feel the heat of the sun on the palms of your hands. Breathe deeply, relax and do not think of anything for five minutes.

2. Walk along the beach and walk in and out of the sea without letting the water come up above your knees.

## What is health?

Enjoying good health is maintaining a dynamic balance among organic functions. It is a way of living biologically; it is the mind that has a powerful influence on our immunity system; it is maintaining an interest in life, a sign of inner youth; it is the state of complete physical, mental and social well-being; it is remaining calm in the face of problems; it is opening up the spiritual dimension of the human being; it is keeping your blood and psyche healthy; it is the coveted desire of living a long and full life. However, why is this desire not easy to achieve? Because our basic energy is not in harmony, in other words, individual, genetic or ancestral energy is not in harmony with the outer or cosmic energy that includes food, water, sun, hygiene, exercise, rest and the world that surrounds us; health is the balance between both energies.

Physical, mental and emotional health depends on cellular purity through purity of blood. We have 50 trillion cells.

**The cell.** The cell is the most fundamental and simplest element of tissues; most metabolic reactions take place (physical, chemical and biological) inside cells and the organism depends on them to maintain its balance (homeostasis). Cells need oxygen, water, nutrients, an even temperature and elimination to function properly.

Electromagnetic activity takes place in cells; they are transmitters, however, their frequency decreases when toxicity affects their metabolism. Matter has two properties: it reflects light and emits light.

There are three types of cells and they have different forms and properties according to their functions:

- Permanent cells: those that last all our life: nerve cells striated muscular fibers.

- Labile cells: those that are constantly renewing themselves: red blood cells, skin cells, etc.

- Stable cells: those that stop multiplying at a certain time during development of the organism, but that multiply again in the event of loss, for example, glandular cells (liver, pancreas, kidneys) and bone cells, cartilaginous cells and smooth muscular fiber cells.

**Tissues:** structures based on groups of cells, generally of the same type, in addition to cellular products and fibers.

**Organs:** formed by one or several tissues that have a specific function, such as the liver, kidneys or lungs.

**Apparatus or systems:** formed by one or several organs grouped in relation to the same organic function, for example, the digestive system.

## HYGIENE BY FASTING

It is recommendable that you see a naturist doctor before fasting. Fasting consists of not taking on any solid food, just liquids, and gives your organism, mind, and emotions the chance to rest. As such, this form of rest is a cure, because it reduces toxicity and gives us the opportunity to rid ourselves of the "junk" food that has accumulated over the years. It also gives us a great opportunity to commence the reversion process in order to recover our health. The circulatory system is cleaned, which improves the heart as it has to work less. Accumulated toxins that have damaged the organism are eliminated when blood is purified.

It is well known that the animal kingdom is wise; it knows what to eat, what to drink, how to live, and when it feels ill it stops eating and eats foliage only, therefore it has always had the wisdom of doing a therapeutic fasting. Even when man is ill, has no appetite or feels nauseous, he insists on eating to "keep his strength up". He eats food that is the most difficult to digest and drinks harmful beverages.

The sensation of revulsion or nausea is produced by the liver or pancreas reacting instinctively when they are too full and when it is difficult for them to digest food. Fasting invigorates and revitalizes the body and gives it the opportunity to activate its defense mechanisms against illness. It is recommendable to fast from the organic, mental, spiritual, economic, cosmetic (rejuvenation), weight reduction, etc., point of view. During and after fasting, the body takes on surprising amounts of energy; it becomes more beautiful and vibrant, in addition to which it releases the ego and turns it into a being that is more sensitive to creation and to itself.

Fasting is a safe way of loosing weight, reducing blood pressure and levels of cholesterol. You should not fast more than three days.

Cellular nutrition does not take place when there are impurities in the body. If they come into contact with cells, cells defend themselves as a fever or some curative crisis to release damaging substances from the organism. The symptoms of curative crisis are: headache, diarrhea, bad breath, catarrh and skin rash. The solution is found in cleanliness of the intestines. If you have fever, apply cold friction on the spinal column and rest as much as you can. In the evening, apply an enema of boiled water with essence of eucalyptus. It is recommendable that you continue fasting with fruit juices or one type of fruit. Eat anything you fancy in moderation so that your organs rest. Fruit nourishes and cleans. Fasting with raw vegetable juice increases the organism's alkalinity and accelerates the healing process. While fasting, drink chamomile tea with bee's honey in order to prevent colic and the desire to eat.

Work on your health, only you can do it!
- Fast intelligently
- Fasting strengthens your will power and character.
- If you fast once a week, you will spend 15% less on food (and loose weight).
- You will save time on both shopping and preparing food.
- When fasting, we discover our true dietary needs and recover our appreciation for the natural flavor of food.
- It is a moral act for those who are hungry, ill, and to ourselves.
- The effect of fasting reaches the very soul of our being.

Note: "… it is recommendable to change gradually from a meat-based diet to a vegetarian-based diet, according to the age of the individual. This will ensure better results because if you change quickly from one diet to the other, the albumin of the tissues will disintegrate and create a state of intoxication due to nitrogen becoming separated from the tissues. This will cause malnutrition, as nitrogen fixes all other materials of the organism".

## Substitute diet: it should be 20% acid and 80% alkaline.

**Alkaline food** (resort to this more frequently):  Lime, carrot, spinach, parsley, cabbage, green beans, potatoes, green chili, pumpkin, corn, avocado, lettuce, beetroot, yoghurt, molasses, maple syrup, grapes, bananas, figs, pears, melons, coconut, nuts, almonds, dates, raisins and prunes.

**Food high in sodium** (resort to these more frequently as they prevent tumors, gallstones and arthritis): celery, chard, spinach, romaine lettuce, beetroot, cabbage, strawberries, pumpkin, potatoes, figs, limes and carrots.

**Food high in potassium** (its deficiency causes problems in the arteries, the heart, and the kidneys): lime, lettuce, beetroot, onion, garlic, red tomatoes, turnip, cabbage, cucumber, cauliflower, brussels sprouts, potatoes, carrots, celery, pumpkin, artichoke, eggplant, broccoli, parsley, basil, ginger, plums, raisins, papaya, grapefruit, banana, fresh fruit, green kidney beans, broad beans, chickpeas, lentils, beans, rice, all cereals, milk whey, egg yolk, soy milk, soy yoghurt, soy oil or safflower oil (a minimum quantity for frying) and dandelion.

| Tap water | Replace with | Distilled, reverse osmosis or magnetic water; 6 to 8 glasses a day. |
|---|---|---|

| | | |
|---|---|---|
| Liquid with meals | Replace with | Drink half an hour before or after |
| Cold liquids | Replace with | Drinks at room temperature |
| Coffee, alcohol, sodas, black tea | Replace with | Herb tea or vegetable or fruit juice. |
| Cow's milk | Replace with | Tofu, soy milk or goat's milk |
| White bread | Replace with | Whole meal bread |
| White flour | Replace with | Whole meal flour |
| White sugar | Replace with | Molasses, bee's honey, maple syrup, brown sugar |
| Cereals without husk | Replace with | Whole meal cereals |
| Fried food | Replace with | Raw or lightly boiled food |
| Canned food | Replace with | Fresh or lightly boiled food |
| Hydrogenated oils | Replace with | Natural oils |

## Incompatibilities

All stages of the natural digestive function (in the mouth, stomach and intestines), produce the enzymes needed for digestion and, at the same time, create disparate elements contrary to the reciprocal effects.

Therefore, incompatibility consists of the incorrect combination of food, bringing about digestive and biochemical problems.

Eat two types of foods with different digestion time at the same meal, for example:

- A fruit that takes two hours to digest with another fruit that takes one hour to digest.

- Starch, digested in an alkaline medium, and protein digested in an acid medium, so starch not digested absorbs pepsin and protein not digested properly, causes slow digestion, putrefaction and fermentation that, in turn, produces alcohol.

- Sugars block the digestion of proteins.

- Two concentrated foods eaten at the same time putrefy and cannot be assimilated.

- When the substance of food nullifies the effects of other foods, for example: Acids and starch, or sweets and fats, or two different sources of starch (rice and potatoes). It is evident that acids annul the action of ptyalin on starches, so eating acid fruit before a meal which has a large quantity of starch is harmful to your health, for example: red tomatoes and vinegar with potatoes and pasta. Excess fat has an adverse effect on gastric secretion, but if you eat a vegetable salad before the meal, the vegetables will absorb the harmful fat. Sugars tend to ferment when consumed in quantity together with food that is affected by the action of gastric juice, for example: cake eaten at the end of a meal produces gas and it is not recommendable to eat bread and butter and jam, as we are accustomed to do.

**Summary:**

- Vegetables rule. Combine well with all food.

- Leguminous food should be combined with green-leaf vegetables.

- Starch does not combine well with fat, protein, sweets, acids and other starches.

- Cooked or raw fruit is compatible with vegetables and other food.

Incompatibilities are not that serious, provided that we follow a few observations:

- Chew slowly and salivate starch, flour, pasta, bread and sweet fruit.

- Do not drink liquid during a meal because it dilutes gastric juices.

- Drink sufficient water between meals and eat at least half a kilogram of fruit a day.

- Take powdered brewing yeast with your food every day or with fruit juice between meals. It includes vitamins of the B group (riboflavin in particular) that help in the assimilation of starch. It is recommendable to add yeast to flour-based recipes.

**Harmful additives** are those mentioned in the label that says "contains" monosodium glutamate, flavoring and artificial coloring, nitrates, BHA, BHT, MSG and substances ending with the letters OSE, such as dextrose.

# COMPATIBILITIES AND INCOMPATIBILITIES

For vegetable proteins if vegetable salad is included it could be used potatoes, rice or millet as garnish

contains no starches:

| | |
|---|---|
| Broccoli | Cabbage |
| Bamboo | Green beans |
| Onions | Turnip |
| Peas | Mushrooms |
| Leeks | Cauliflower |
| Eggplant | Brussels sprout |
| Carrots | White Salsify |
| Sprouts | Cucumber |
| Chayote | |

Green Leaves:

| | |
|---|---|
| Endive | Beet leaves |
| Spinach | Carrot leaves |
| Parsley | Celery leaves |
| Chard | Dandelion |
| Lettuce | Watercress |

Fresh fruits are refreshing for the digestive system and excellent to avoid the effort of delicate intestines

| | |
|---|---|
| Hazelnuts | Beans |
| Walnuts | Soya beans |
| Chestnuts | Dry peas |
| Almonds | Legumes |
| Peanuts | Lentils |
| Pistachios | Chickpeas |
| Pine nuts | Milk |
| Figs | Curd |
| Dry fruits | Yogurt |
| Olives | Cheese |
| Amaranth | Grains |

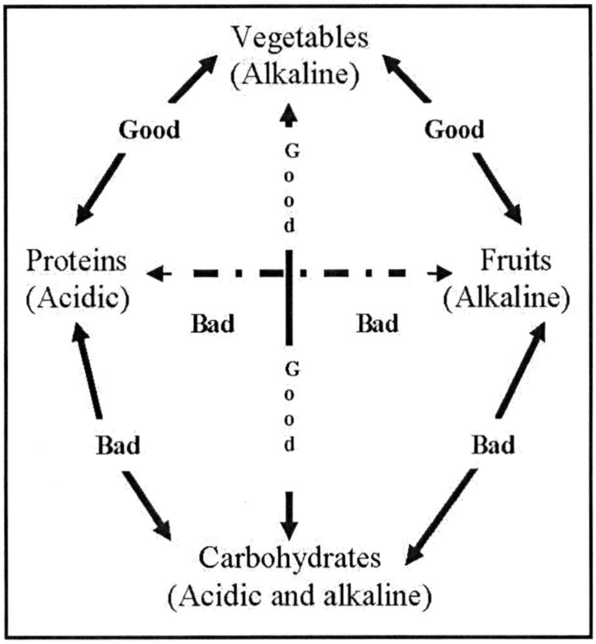

Vegetables
(Alkaline)
Good
Good
Good
Proteins
(Acidic)
Fruits
(Alkaline)
Bad
Bad
Good
Bad
Bad
Carbohydrates
(Acidic and alkaline)


Sweet fruits:

| | |
|---|---|
| Dates | Bananas |
| Figs | Dry fruits |
| Raisins | Sugar cane |
| Mangoes (all) | Cantaloupes |
| Watermelon | |

Semi-acidic fruits:

| | |
|---|---|
| Berries | Orange |
| Bilberry | Grapefruit |
| Cherry | Pineapple |
| Blackberry | Pear |
| Plum | Papaya |
| Apricot | Haw fruit |
| Peaches | Grape |
| Mango | Quince |
| Apple | Guava |

Acidic fruits:

| | |
|---|---|
| Orange | Strawberry |
| Lime | Pomegrate |
| Tomato | Red Currant |
| Tamarind | Mandarin |

Yogurt and dry fruits or bananas are well combined

Don't mix two different types of proteins.

Whole grains, oleaginous and sprouts are a good source of proteins.

Vegetables:

| | |
|---|---|
| Artichoke | Potatoes |
| Chestnuts | Corn |
| Pumpkin | Pea |
| Dry peas | Avocado |
| Beetroot | Banana |

Whole Cereals:

| | |
|---|---|
| Oat | Barley |
| Rice | Rye |
| Wheat | Millet |

Bread
Cakes
Pastas
Candies

Mix acidic fruits only with acidic fruits and cantaloupes only with cantaloupes

# A GLANCE AT BREAKFAST AND DINNER

Take your time when having breakfast; you will lead a more contended life if you feel better.

Breakfast is the first meal of the day and not having breakfast can often cause serious stomach problems such as colitis, gastritis, peptic ulcers, and other health problems.

The level of sugar in the blood decreases at the beginning of the day due to not having taken on any food for a long time, so it is important to have breakfast. When the brain is thinking it needs glucose to produce energy and begins to use fats stored in reserve. As this is not an efficient system, our performance reduces and we feel bad tempered or dizzy. This is also due to the fact that two-thirds of the nervous system uses glucose (sugar) to function correctly. Drinking coffee only causes a sense of anxiety which the organism gets used to.

Give yourself a treat in the morning with a breakfast that contains carbohydrates (cereal, bread, honey, fresh or dry fruit, etc), proteins (eggs, yoghurt, cottage cheese or beans) and all those nutrients that contain the twenty-two amino acids. Yoghurt contains eighteen amino acids and the rest may be found in royal jelly, honey, pollen, raisins, almonds, pumpkin seeds, oats, etc., and seasonal fruit. Before breakfast, drinking hot tea made from herbs, horsetail, dandelion, chamomile, or hot water with lime juice (before bathing) purifies the kidneys.

Breakfast should be suitable for each person according to their physical activity, age, sex, weight, height, etc.

It is recommendable to preferably eat the same cereal at breakfast that you had at dinner. For example:

The soup on menu No. 5 is made from oats, so the cereal eaten at breakfast on the same day should be oats, with fruit, raisins or prunes or nuts to taste. Oats should be eaten raw and soaked (the organism assimilates it better) or cooked to taste, with cinnamon, cardamom or anise and honey made from unrefined sugar.

A good breakfast provides you energy, vitamins, minerals, etc. For example:

- Fresh seasonal fruit of your choice, cereal and/or prunes soaked in water.

- Fruit, yoghurt with bran, nuts, grain or muesli, and honey.

- Fruit, oat rice or barley cereal, and honey made from unrefined sugar.

- Fruit, a sandwich made of whole meal, black or rye bread, with fresh cheese, etc.

- A drink made from carrots, beetroot, milk, pine nut, sesame seed, dates or apples.

Around midday: an alfalfa juice with pineapple, or a citric juice with alfalfa tablets or brewer's yeast tablets.

**DINNER:** It is suggested something light, for example:

- A vegetable salad that may include a moderate quantity of the midday soup.

- Fruit and a glass of almond milk (blend a glass of water, 7-10 almonds and honey).

- A combination of apples, lettuce, celery and wheat germ that will clean your arteries and improve your skin, nails and hair.

## NUTRITION, VITAL FOR ELDERLY PEOPLE

Why do we get old?

Researchers say that cells reproduce themselves and that old age is brought on by a failure in "quality control" at the time of division (mitosis). This failure is what causes illness in old age. Defective cells should be detained before they reproduce and be separated before they enter the mitosis stage.

Physiological functions or metabolic processes, together with physical activity, decrease as we get older. There is a major decrease in the consumption of calories and other nutrients, so consumption of fat and empty calories should be reduced substantially and more nutritional food, such as whole meal, cereal should be eaten, along with all types of fresh and raw or lightly steamed fruit and vegetables, wheat germ, juice and pure water. There is also a major deficiency of certain minerals such as iron, calcium, and protein and vitamin D and other vitamins, such as folic acid (B9), caused by stress during period of illness. Antibiotics change or affect the flora of the small intestine, reducing microbial production of riboflavin (B2), biotin and vitamin K.

The organism of an old person or an ill person should be looked after, not only by taking proper medication, but also by avoiding stressful exercise, chills, and scrupulously eating the proper food, which should be healthy and bland and not include irritating foods, and contain as little fat as possible. Canned food, too many sweets and chocolates should be avoided (because they prevent the assimilation of calcium), along with peanuts and alcohol. It is also important to eat at a specific time, slowly, and to chew all food carefully.

The solution to enjoying a long and healthy life is to lead a healthy life by restricting the intake of empty calories and providing your organism with high quantities of calories at breakfast, as well as taking on antioxidant supplements and taking light exercise, such as walking.

Simple recommendations:

- Adapt your diet.

- Have a set time for eating and eat nutritional food between meals, such as juices.

- Appetite decreases with age, so light and nutritional food should be eaten, but more frequently.

- An energy-giving food is recommended (see bee's pollen).

## WHAT TO EAT?

1. Fruit

2. Garden produce and vegetables

3. Whole meal grain

4. Oleaginous products

5. Products of animal origin

The **Vegetable Kingdom** provides us fruit, vegetables, leguminous products, cereals, roots, oleaginous products, all rich in carbohydrates, vitamins, minerals and amino acids. The composition of these elements changes according to place, condition of the earth, weather and amount of rainfall.

Raw food produced organically in fertile soil is vital and has a powerful preventive effect, because it contains enzymes, live organic atoms, sugars and flours easy to assimilate. The carbohydrates that they contain provide calories, cellulose and are an excellent source of energy and reserves.

Much of the importance of raw vegetable food is that the vitamins and minerals that they contain act as structural molecules that are indispensable for the functioning of our body's many enzymes. Enzymes are the very heart of life: they facilitate digestion of food and their absorption in the blood.

Vegetables are not only nutritional, but also have therapeutic qualities that have been known since ancient times. They are also used as medical poultice. Recent research shows that there is a direct association between a vegetable and fruit-based diet and good health. Researchers have found that vegetables include a group of nutrients called phytochemicals or phytonutrients, substances that give plants their color and taste. They are biologically active substances and are important in protecting us against illness.

Some include flavonoids (citrics) indoles (cabbage), saponines (legumes), genesteins (soy beans), licopenes, ellagic acids, etc. Nature has thousands of phytonutrients.

Researchers acknowledge that eating fruit, vegetables, grains and legumes reduce the risk of many illnesses. The preventive effect is mainly due to antioxidants, such as vitamins A and C, which trap the free radicals that may damage DNA cells and develop tumors. Beta carotenes are nearly always the precursors of vitamin A and are found in orange and yellow-colored fruits and vegetables. Vitamin C is found in abundance in citric fruit.

Food is the substance that we give our body; it is the fuel that gives energy to it and that keeps us alive. Food is light and color. When vegetables grow they absorb sunlight (photosynthesis) and turn it into colors. When we eat any food, the organism breaks it down and once again turns it into light and color. "Light and color act as the link between idea and form, conscience and supraconscience (Inner Self)…"

Sustenance is what we eat. Nutrients are the substances received by cells. For example, combine legumes and cereals that provide complete protein (the combination of leguminous products and cereals include minerals, vitamins, carbohydrates, fats and fibers) more garden produce and fruits and your organism will receive excellent nourishment.

They contain amino acids that the body does not produce: carrots, bananas, brussels sprouts, cabbage, cauliflower, corn, cucumber, eggplant, peas, potatoes, red tomatoes, pumpkin, nuts, sesame seeds, sunflower seeds and peanuts.

Eating is an art and a science. Healthy eating is also a pleasurable experience! Vegetables not only provide nutrients, but many also have therapeutic qualities.

Therapeutic information given regarding vegetable based food should be supervised by medical practitioners or naturist therapists.

But remember that you have an old ally in natural food free of synthetic substances.

## BASIC DAILY DIET

- 80% fruit and vegetables.

- 20% whole meal grain, oleaginous products, yoghurt and honey.

- 8 glasses of water or juices, including herb tea.

Less frequently (three times a week) eat mayonnaise, oils, potatoes, herbs, eggs, cheese, sweets, etc.

Eliminate the following: meat, alcohol, sweets, cakes, refined products, white sugar, pasta, fried or canned food and carbonated drinks (sodas).

# 1. Fruit

Nature has been truly generous in terms of quantity, color, shapes, aromas and flavors, as far as fruits are concerned, all of which are adapted to different conditions of land and climate. Fruit carries out very important functions, such as alkalinizing blood to counteract excess acidity produced by some food such as eggs, cereals and meat. The function of fruit is to clean, nourish and heal the organism.

Seasonal fruit has its maximum biological value when picked ripe. Fruit is picked unripe to be transported from one place to another, distributed and sold, and it loses part of its properties.

Fruit includes all nutritive elements that man needs to live. We should enjoy them and acquaint ourselves with them, but eat them on an individual basis.

It is recommendable to eat fruit unpeeled and to chew the pips. Fruit contains soluble fiber that helps to reduce cholesterol, and insoluble fiber that helps to prevent constipation. For ideal assimilation, it is better to eat just one type of fruit at the same meal, or no more than two.

Cantaloupe and watermelon are better eaten on their own and if you blend the pips with water you will get a delicious *horchata*

Fresh fruit and juices provide a large part of the vitamin C we need. Fruit with most vitamin C includes: limes, oranges, tangerines, grapefruit, strawberries, kiwi fruit and guavas. Acidic fruits are high in antioxidants, such as vitamin C and bioflavonoid that help to protect us against chronic and degenerative diseases such as heart attack, hypertension and cancer (clinically proven).

Dark-yellow or orange fruits contain beta-carotene that protect us against free radicals (precursors of some types of cancer), these fruits including mangoes, cantaloupes, peaches and apricots.

**The following information is just an example of the wide variety that nature gives us, its nutritive value and its therapeutic use.**

**Bilberry.** Still grows wild. Grows in clumps. High in sugars, amino acids, vitamins, mineral salts and acids, so it is an excellent source of nutrition in a balanced proportion and provides Vitamin C.

**Therapeutic indication**: Helps to eliminate toxins and uric acid. Helps the respiratory system. Useful for intestinal, circulatory and respiratory disorders. Invigorates the digestive system. Useful against diarrhea and kills infectious viruses. Excellent for the prostate gland.

**Sugar cane.** This plant is pure sugar (carbohydrates). The juice provides lots of energy, is high in nutrients and is easy to assimilate. Contains sucrose, minerals and vitamins in the correct proportion.

**Therapeutic indication:** It is diuretic and refreshing. It is an effective anti-acid. It reduces inflammation of the stomach and the connecting organs and relieves gastric or duodenal ulcers. Cooked sugar cane helps to alleviate problems of the respiratory, urinary and jaundice. Naturist doctors highly recommend sugar-cane juice during fasting for pulmonary tuberculosis.

**Capulin cherry.** Highly nutritive. Contains a balanced quantity of proteins and carbohydrates; minerals: iron, calcium, sodium, potassium, phosphorous, manganese, magnesium, sulfur, silica and chlorine. Vitamins: A, B and C.

**Therapeutic indication:** Invigorates the nervous system and the brain, Activates circulation. Excellent for problems related to the respiratory system, stomach, intestine, kidneys, liver, gallbladder, anemia, obesity, arteriosclerosis and rheumatism, and helps to relieve constipation.

**Cherries.** A delicious semi-acidic berry with high nutritional value.

**Therapeutic indication:** Detoxifies the organism and replenishes minerals. Activates renal secretion. Cherry stalk tea is a powerful diuretic, as is the fruit itself. It is recommended for people suffering from rheumatism, arthritis, arteriosclerosis and gastric disorders.

**Apricot.** Slightly acidic and very tasty. Very nutritional and contains beta carotene.

**Therapeutic indication:** Increases red blood cells, therefore it is good for anemia-related problems. An excellent reconstituting element; excellent for the skin and hair; helps to alleviate constipation, anemia, nervous excitement and retention of liquids. Recommended for children and convalescents to improve their health. Known to prevent cancer, particularly lung cancer.

**Plum.** A wide variety, tasty and semi-acidic. Contains the following minerals: iron, phosphorous, calcium, magnesium, manganese, potassium, and sodium, plus vitamins B1, B2, C and A ,the latter being the most abundant. Easily-digestible sugars, cellulose and alkalinizing acids. Plums have a high proportion of carbohydrates.

**Therapeutic indications.** Helps healing bronchial disorders, rheumatism and arteriosclerosis. It is diuretic, detoxifying and decongests the liver. It provides physical and intellectual energy. They are slightly laxative and ease constipation. Plums are laxative and high in fiber, it is also a type of natural aspirin. Drinking plum juice while fasting helps you to remain healthy.

**Coconut.** A wonderful plant, all of which may be used to benefit our health. Its milk is the best there is: high in essential amino acids, lots of minerals, vitamin C and complex B vitamins; high in phosphate-based substances that invigorate the nervous system. It is one of the healthiest forms of nourishment.

**Therapeutic Indication:** Coconut milk is excellent for reconstituting the entire organism. It is diuretic and helps to relieve constipation and weakness in general. Improves digestion and eliminates parasites. When fasting, drink two to three cups a day for three weeks. May be used for dehydration. Coconut pulp taken during fasting removes intestinal worms. Disinfects, purifies and mineralizes. Recommended for physical and mental exhaustion. Eliminates uric acid. Natural coconut oil applied locally relieves hemorrhoids and helps to prevent and treat sunburn and certain skin infections.

**Dates.** Have all indispensable nutrients for the human body. Pleasant and easy to digest, even for the most delicate stomachs. Its minerals include: calcium, potassium and phosphorous, and it has a good balance of vitamins A, B, C and D, pectin and starch; high in carbohydrates in the form of glucose and laevulose, so it provides lots of energy.

**Therapeutic Indication**: Of great help to the respiratory system, better when taking as a syrup (boil dates in water). Serves as a laxative; helps to prevent cancer of the pancreas; useful for intoxication, hepatitis and circulative disorders. It is said that the stone crushed in capsules taken in micro-dose helps against tuberculosis, increases appetite and decreases diarrhea.

**Peaches**. There are several types: hard (peaches) and soft (*priscos*) Should be eaten ripe. They are nutritional and give energy; rich in pro-vitamin A, and vitamins C, B1, B2, B3, B5, and B9; minerals include sodium, potassium, calcium, manganese, magnesium, iron, phosphorous, sulfur, copper, chloride and zinc.

**Therapeutic Indication**: When eaten in large quantities, detoxifies the organism; gently stimulates gastric juices; slightly laxative and helps in difficult digestion; slightly diuretic; useful for glandular problems, muscular tiredness and general weakness; improves the blood. Peel may be applied to the skin to detoxify it, open pores and reaffirm tissue. The pulp invigorates and revitalizes the nervous and reproductive system; strengthens the structural system; supports liver and spleen functions, and helps prevent lung cancer. Juice drunk during fasting relieves sore throat, lung problems, constipation and removes intestinal parasites. The flowers on tea have a sedative effect.

**Raspberries**. A fruit that still grows wild. A delicious semi-acidic berry with high nutritive value that should always be part of your diet.

Therapeutic Indication: Mineralizes and detoxifies. Helps in problems of cellulites, constipation and lack of appetite. Suitable for people suffering from diabetes. Provides levulose and vitamin C.

**Strawberry**. A delicious and lovely fruit of the berry family that includes well- balanced nutritional elements. Should be eaten fresh and ripe, not as a sweet. Do not mix with alcohol, oil, vinegar or vegetables. It is an excellent source of vitamin C and A, all vitamins of the group B, B3, E, K, and beta carotene. Acts as an antioxidant due to its content of antocianines and polyphenols. High in minerals such as iron, phosphorous, potassium, magnesium, manganese, sulfur, bromide and iodine, and has a high content of salicylic acid. Proteins, carbohydrates, fibers, pigments, acids and fat.

**Therapeutic Indication**:  Acts as a powerful regenerator and purifier of the blood; alkalinizes and mineralizes. It is a great hepatic regenerator; slightly laxative and diuretic. Contains special nutrients for diabetics in convalescence; useful for n afflictions of the nervous system, the urinary system, the respiratory system and the gallbladder; useful for arterial hypertension due to its low content of sodium and its high content of potassium. Anti-cancerous. Salicylic acid is good for the liver, kidneys and articulations, but do not take in cases of intolerance to aspirin. People who tend to form oxalate renal gallstones should eat strawberries in moderation due to their content of oxalic acid. In cases of gout, arthritis and rheumatism eat half a kilogram a day. When applied externally they cure chilblains. The legend says that they prolong life. The small spots on the fruit contribute to intestine elimination functions.

**Blackcurrant**. Tradition says that it is an excellent elixir of life that keeps you young and healthy. Has a high content of vitamins C and P.

**Therapeutic Indication**: Excellent for reconstituting. Leaf stalks are excellent for rheumatism. Diuretic.

**Guava**. There are several varieties with yellow, white or red pulp. It has a high content of vitamin C, retained in its dry state, vitamins A, B1, B2, salts, minerals, carbohydrates, protein, and citric, tannic, and malic acids, and mucilage.

**Therapeutic Indication**: The unripe fruit is astringent and good for diarrhea; ripe fruit is slightly laxative.

When eaten during fasting, it removes intestinal parasites. Useful for diarrhea in children and inflammation of the legs; has a rapid effect if eaten three times a day.

**Figs**. Very complete in nutrients so it is ideal for dieting. An excellent source of energy (fresh: 60 calories for every 100 grams; dry: 243 calories for every 100 grams). Eat when ripe. It has a variety of vitamins, but in small quantities, the high proportion of which are those of group B, mainly found in dry figs. Have lots of minerals: potassium, calcium, phosphorous, magnesium and iron. Ideal for children's school lunch, together with nuts or almonds. The "Breva" is a variety of the fig.

**Therapeutic Indication**: Facilitates expectoration in case of hacking, dry coughs, with better results if taken as a fig, date and raisin syrup. You may also boil 30 grams of dry leaves in one liter of water and then stand for fifteen minutes, strain and drink one cup three times a day. Eating fresh figs during fasting has a laxative effect; applied as a poultice it reduces spots, abscesses, inflammation and injuries (dry figs cut in half, cooked in milk, strained, shredded and applied to the affected area.) May be used to treat nervous asthenia. Apply the milk of fig stalks with cotton wool on corns and warts twice a day until they dry.

**Kiwi fruit.** An excellent source of vitamin C and other nutrients.

**Therapeutic Indication**: Helps the respiratory system, mainly the lymphatic system.

**Mangoes**. There are many varieties with a pleasant and sweet taste. Should be eaten ripe raw, not green. It has an acidifying if eaten in excess. Contains vitamin C and B complex vitamin; high in beta-carotene (pro-vitamin A); rich in minerals: calcium, potassium and phosphorous; carbohydrates, proteins and citric, gallic, tannic and tartaric acids.

**Therapeutic Indication**: Purifies the organism, replenishes minerals and purifies the blood. Reinforces the nervous system; useful for cerebral fatigue, insomnia and depression; have a laxative effect. Helps in gastrointestinal problems and those of the respiratory system. Eating manila mango helps the respiratory system. All varieties are good for neuralgic afflictions and rheumatism, when eaten with strawberries. Regularizes menstruation, acts on the reproductive system and increases women's sexuality. Leaves may be cooked in water and when gargled helps to eliminate pyorrhea, set loose teeth and relieve toothache and sore throat.

**Apples**. There are hundreds of varieties available all year round. Apples have been eaten for centuries and have always been appreciated for their nutritional and medicinal qualities. Tasty and easy to digest; should be eaten with the peel and chew well to extract all their nutrients. Contain proteins, cellulose, sugars, including dextrose, levulose and saccharose, gums, pectin, protopectin, pentosones, and organic, citric, lactic, malic, tannic, and other acids. Minerals: phosphorous, potassium, sodium, iron, calcium, magnesium, copper, chlorine, manganese, sulfur and zinc; low in vitamin C and complex B. The peel is rich in cellulose, vitamin C, iron, and phosphorous. When eaten before meals, salts and acids disinfect the digestive system, thus improving digestion; when eaten after meals, they ensure correct gastrointestinal functioning, and when eaten at evening meals they protect the teeth and gums. A full meal for children in school comprises: apple, nuts or almonds and raisins; it gives them energy and it is healthy for the brain. It is an excellent restorative food.

**Therapeutic Indication**: An excellent physical and intellectual tonic for the nervous system and structural system. Strengthens the digestive-intestinal system; useful for diarrhea, arthritis, rheumatism and gout; reduces inflammation of the kidneys and the bladder and treats infections of the respiratory system; stimulates and regularizes insulin; useful for proper functioning of the heart; reduces cholesterol and high blood pressure; anemia and demineralization. Pectin stimulates the intestine and absorbs gases and toxins, purifying the organism. Potassium facilitates elimination of uric acid. Includes anti-cancerous agent (antioxidants). Useful for the skin, and infections of the liver and spleen; stabilizes sugar; stimulates the appetite. When cooked, helps against constipation, due to its high content of fiber. Children with gastrointestinal infections should eat them unripe raw and shredded for three days. The peel boiled in water helps digestion, strengthens the bronchi and invigorates the organism. Apples are recommended against any illness. Having an apple, celery, lettuce and wheat germ salad for supper helps keep your arteries, nails and skin healthy and makes the skin more attractive.

**Apple vinegar** is an excellent fermented juice that contains yeast and essential minerals. It purifies and refreshes. It is an excellent antiseptic for the digestive system and removes bacteria.

It contains malic acid, indispensable for digestion, reduces intestinal fermentation, keeps the circulatory system healthy and helps you to relax. High in potassium, it is necessary for muscular activity. Its acidity compensates the organism's acid/alkaline balance. Hippocrates recommended it diluted in water to be taken for afflictions such as asthma, arthritis and digestion. Prepare the vinegar with one liter of water, a cone of unrefined sugar (piloncillo) and three finely diced apples with the core removed. Leave for seven days, strain and refrigerate.

**Cantaloupe.** Contains minerals: phosphorous, calcium, potassium and iron; small quantities of vitamins A, B1, B2 and C, plus a high amount of alkalinizing water, but its nutritional value is low. It should not be eaten with watermelon, oleaginous fruit, oils, dairy products or vegetables. Combines well with sweet and dry fruit and honey.

**Therapeutic Indication**: Its mineral nature helps to detoxify and rejuvenate tissue. An excellent laxative and appetizer: it is diuretic; useful against gastric acidity, spasmodic constipation, gout, rheumatism, and helps the liver and kidneys. As it stimulates gastric juices, it is recommendable to eat it before meals; eating after meals usually causes digestive problems.

**Quince**. Quince pulp is excellent against vomiting and diarrhea, but only if the fruit was picked after the first frost, if not, it has the contrary effect. The pips may used to make a tea that helps to calm hemorrhoids, and treat breast fissures and mouth infections.

**Oranges**. Originate in China. There are many types of citric fruits: sweet and sour oranges, grapefruit, lemon, royal lemon and tangerine. The tree provides us fruit, pips, flowers, leaves, bark and root. Fruit should be eaten ripe and it is good to eat the white part of the peel as it contains vitamin C and bioflavonoid. High in vitamin C and bioflavonoid (vitamin P), and in vitamins A, B1, B2, B3, B5, B6, A, E, H, K; minerals include potassium, phosphorous, magnesium, calcium, chloride, sulfur, sodium, iron, manganese, copper, bromide, and zinc. Calories. Has high energy value. The skin of each section contains riboflavin (vitamin B2). Glutathione.

**Therapeutic Indication**: It is anti-scorbutic; has detoxifying properties that remove harmful or toxic substances from the organism; decongests; useful for gastrointestinal infections and constipation of the stomach; purifies the kidneys, liver and spleen; dissolves uric acid; prevents and corrects problems of the respiratory system. Contains all known types of natural cancer inhibitors, particularly stomach cancer and breast cancer. Useful for bleeding and inflamed gums; helps to alleviate physical and mental depression. Dry oranges are excellent for purifying the liver and the gallbladder. Leaves eaten with boiled pips are excellent for coughs, and improve digestion, calm palpitations of the heart, and alleviate headaches and insomnia. According to Professor Capo, they cure diabetes, syphilis, cancer and gonorrhea.

**Grapefruit** facilitate the removal of fat. They are nutritious, purifying and have diuretic properties. Tea made from peel combats flatulence. The white part is high in pectin and soluble fiber that protect the heart. Drinking orange juice and grapefruit juice helps to prevent heart attack and angina pectoris.

**Papaya**. Delicious and refreshing with low nutritive value. Contains calories, carbohydrates and vitamins C, A, B1, B2, B3 and D; minerals: calcium, magnesium, potassium, iron and sodium; low in tannic and malic acids; high in proteolytic enzymes that help digestion of proteins, such as papain, vegetable pepsin that separates proteins into amino acids, arginine that helps masculine fertility; fibrin helps in the coagulation process, and carpaine helpful to the heart. Papaya enzymes act on acidic, neutral or alkaline media and it is useful for treating gastric ulcers.

**Therapeutic Indication**: Purifying. It is a gentle laxative and anthelmintic. Useful for digestive and glandular disorders and rheumatism; recovers bacteria which helps the organism; helps the liver and the gallbladder; reduces cholesterol. Enzymes in the pips improve digestion and prevent or remove gas from the intestine, eat just one or two. Causes menstruation. The dry pips crushed and served with bee's honey removes intestinal worms. Eat during fasting for five days: ten pips for children weighing over 10 kgs., and twenty pips for adults. The **leaves** remove blotches from the skin and stains from clothes: just scrub them against fresh stains before washing. Tea made from leaves helps the respiratory system. **External use:** the inner peel helps to cure skin wounds and may be used for beauty treatment. The **pulp** reduces inflammation and is useful for sunburn. By making a cut in the **green fruit** attached to the papaya, you may extract a milky juice that when drunk fresh is a good anthelmintic and harmless.

**Pears**. There are many varieties. It is a tasty fruit; the sweeter the more nutritious and easily and quickly digestible. Eat unripe with the peel. Contains soluble fiber, rich in iodine; contains calcium, magnesium, phosphorous, potassium, beta carotene, folic acid, and peptin that helps peristalsis and to eliminate toxins. May replace apples due to their similar nutritive properties.

**Therapeutic Indication**: Excellent for purifying and replenishing minerals; a light laxative. Helps to remove cholesterol and cellulites; it is diuretic. It has a regulatory action on the intestinal function. Sugar is found in the form of levulose, so it can be eaten by diabetics. Alleviates and improves prostate problems; useful for cystitis, constipation, high pressure and during convalescence. Infused leaves help to reduce inflammation of the bladder and urinary lithiasis.

**Pineapple**. A very tasty fruit with a thick and juicy pulp. It should be eaten ripe and before meals so as to help digestion. For people with sensitive teeth, rinse the mouth with baking soda dissolved in water. Contains vitamins, a good amount of vitamins B1, B3, B5, B9, A and C, and the following mineral salts: calcium, magnesium, potassium, phosphorous, iodine, chloride, sulfur, sodium, iron and copper. Malic and citric acids predominate. Anasia, principle active element in the digestive process. Contains bromelin, a fermenting agent that acts as proteolitic enzyme with very energetic digestive properties.

**Therapeutic Indication**: Eat fresh. An excellent neuro-cerebral tonic; it has antiviral and antibacterial properties. Acts as an appetizer, refreshes the digestive system and stimulates gastric secretion. It is detoxifying, diuretic and nutritive. Useful for dyspepsia; reduces inflammation of the stomach and intestine and helps to heal intestinal ulcers; useful for disorders of the liver and the gallbladder and may help to ease painful menstruation; excellent for arthritis, gout, anemia and arteriosclerosis; functions as a dynamic agent in the pancreas; useful for diabetes; helps to dissolve mucus. The juice is slightly antiseptic and may be used to ease throat problems and bronchitis. Eaten when fasting helps to treat constipation and intestinal gas.

**Bananas**. A tasty fruit available all year round. It should be eaten ripe, but not over ripe or under ripe, so as to make full use of its fructose and levulose. Contain proteins, carbohydrates, calories and malic, tannic, gallic, and peptic acids; vitamins A, B1, B2, B3, K and C; minerals: iron, sodium, calcium, traces of iodine, manganese and zinc, although rich in phosphorous and potassium and other nutrients that the nervous system and the entire organism need.

**Therapeutic Indication**: Revitalize the nervous system; useful for the urinary system, tiredness and growth; a major source of muscular energy; prevents ulcers; strengthens the gastric lining against ulcers due to their high content of pectin; eliminate toxic metals in the organism; help to prevent constipation, hemorrhoids, gastritis and diarrhea. Excellent for people with hypertension, gout or cardiac disorders. Reduce the level of cholesterol; have an antibiotic action; anti-scorbutic and invigorating. Of great energetic and nutritive value and recommendable at any age. Bananas are digested in the mouth, so salivate well when eating. As bananas are very feculent food, they should be eaten on their own. They satisfy the stomach and help you to eat less. Cause digestive problems when eaten as a dessert.

**Watermelon**. Similar properties to those of melon. It has a high quantity of physiological water that cleans the organism of impurities. High quantity of antioxidant and anti-cancerous compounds. Glutathione. It should be eaten ripe and on its own, preferably before meals. Indigestible as a dessert. Its Pips are rich in vitamin E and may be used to make a drink, mixing with the pulp and then straining.

**Therapeutic Indication**: Energetic and refreshing. Reduces inflammation of mucus and prevents the formation of mucus. It is an excellent diuretic. Increases the potential value of red blood cells; purifies the blood; antibacterial; cleans the liver; alleviates intestinal gas; useful for hypertension and fever; has anticoagulant properties (the white part contains vitamin K). It should not be eaten with melon, dairy products, vegetables or oleaginous products.

**Tamarind**. Its excessive acidity decreases the large quantity of sugars in its pulp. Contains vitamin C and B complex, mineral salts; citric and malic acids; pepsin, potassium, tartrate acid (cream of tartar) predominates and has a laxative effect. Pips are high in protein, fat and other nutrients. Is easily digestible, has high energetic value and a good taste. To remove the peel, toast and cook them just like legumes.

**Therapeutic Indication**: Purifies and is diuretic. Useful for problems of the digestive system. Has a purging effect if you eat more than 100 grams.

**Haw fruit**. It is delicious when ripe; nutritive and easy to digest. Increases calories when prepared as a syrup, sweet jelly or preserve.

**Therapeutic Indication**: Useful for disorders of the respiratory system, the bronchi and coughs, take haw fruit syrup. Leaves prepared as a tea helps the urinary system and is diuretic. The root decreases glucose in the blood and urine and is useful for diabetes. It is more potent diuretic than the leaves (45 per liter) and is useful for all kidney infections.

**Prickly pear**. A tasty fruit with lots of water, glucose and cellulose. The intestine may become blocked if the pips are eaten in large quantities. Prepare a delicious juice by liquefying it with water and then straining. Most of its properties are concentrated in the fruit and contains minerals, vitamins, proteins, fats, calories, nitrogenous matter and organic acids.

**Therapeutic Indication**: Useful for respiratory, renal, liver, pancreatic, prostate and arthritic disorders, and diarrhea; helps the circulatory system. Drinking prickly pear juice during fasting will replace physical and mental tiredness, thanks to its high content of sugar.

**Grapes**. The "queen" of fruits, known as the fruit of life. Its abundant dynamic water is of high biological value and one of the best sources of nutrition for the human body. Eat ripe, fresh and with the skin, as it contains vitamins, cellulose and tartaric acid (chew well). Preferably eat on their own and not as a dessert. Contain a high quantity of vitamin C, potassium and manganese. High content of vitamins A and B; minerals: iron, calcium, phosphorous, manganese, sodium, iodine and arsenic; histidine, essential amino acid for children's growth. Organic acids: tartaric, malic, citric, tannic, gallic, salicylic and succinic. Includes elements such as lecithin, thyroxine, lencine and quercetine, and levulose, fructose and glucose (900 calories per kilo) easy to assimilate. Juice is extracted by liquefying grapes with a little water and then straining.

**Therapeutic Indication**: Revitalizes and fortifies muscular tissue; excellent support for the immunity system; helps to reconstitute the organism; it is antibacterial and antiviral; purifies the blood and tissues due to its alkalinizing properties; acts as a laxative and a tonic in the digestive process, facilitating the formation of pepsin. It is diuretic and alleviates weakness, colds and arthritis. Decongests the liver and biliary tracts; helps to prevent myocardial infarctions and arteriosclerosis. Red grapes contain a high quantity of antioxidants and anti-cancerous compounds. Blood may be transformed totally by just eating grapes, improving the organism's health and vitality. It is called "vegetable milk" due to its constitution which is similar to that of mother's milk. Raisins have lost some of their properties but have energetic value and are excellent for the respiratory system.

**Sapodilla fruit**. The pulp is very soft when the fruit is ripe and it is easy to digest. Contains glucose, sacchrose, pectin, starch and calories. There are many varieties of this fruit, such as mamey, small sapodilla, *domingo* sapodilla, *cabello* sapodilla, etc, Everything on the tree may be used: the trunk, leaves, and pips, from which oil is extracted and gum is extracted from the bark.

**Therapeutic Indication**: It is useful for calming rheumatic pain and is a natural sedative for the nervous system.

**Black sapodilla fruit**. The pulp is soft when ripe and is easy to digest. Contains protein, cellulose, fats and gums that protect the stomach, as well as sacchrose, glucose, albuminoids and vitamins A, B1, B2, B3.

**Therapeutic Indication**: Helps digestion and gastritis.

**Blackberry**. A very tasty and semi-acidic fruit that should be eaten ripe. Contains a high quantity of nutrients.

**Therapeutic Indication**: Useful for afflictions such as cystitis, flu, rheum, fever and rickets.

# 2. GARDEN PRODUCE.

**Vegetables and garden produce.** The term "garden produce" includes a wide variety of food. Parts of vegetables and garden produce that can be eaten include: leaves, stems, bulbs, roots and even flowers, and another parts in small quantities may be used as a condiment. The most commonly eaten vegetables are: chard, garlic, celery, artichokes, beetroot, eggplant, cabbage, watercress, broccoli, pumpkins, onions, chives, peas, cauliflower, endives, asparagus, spinach, green beans, lettuce, potatoes, cucumbers, peppers, leeks, radishes, red tomatoes, green tomatoes, turnips, yucca, carrots, etc.

Vegetables constitute a nutritive food due to the large variety of tasty options they offer for all types of dishes. Uncooked they contain all the nutrients that the body needs, and replenish minerals. They contain chlorophyll that has an alkalinizing effect. They are composed of nearly 90% water, they contain dissolved vitamins and are very rich in minerals. They also contain cellulose that helps the peristaltic movement of intestine. **Vegetables** build the organism and are a delight that you will never tire of. You should always have them on your table.

**Root vegetables** grow under the soil, for example, potatoes, yucca and others. It seems that this type of growth is a strategy of the vegetable kingdom in order to bear low temperatures at high altitude. Root vegetables are rich in starch, with an average calorific content but a high quantity of vitamin B3 (niacin), no vitamin D, little protein and a few other nutrients.

You should wash, brush and disinfect vegetables in water with salt and lime, or vinegar, for one hour and wash with purified water. Cook them at the very last moment. Steamed or in a little boiling water is the best way of conserving vegetables' minerals and vitamins. Use this water for soup. Carrots, beetroot and radish **leaves** are of great biological value. After washing the leaves, immerse them in hot water, never cold water, and cook.

### The following information is just an example of the nutritive value of some of the vegetables that Mother Nature has given us.

**Olives**. Normally eaten green and pickled, when they have very little nutritive value. You may extract oil from them when ripe, commonly known as olive oil that has a high nutritive value.

**Therapeutic Indication**: Natural olive oil is an excellent antacid, a smooth laxative and lubricates the intestine; stimulates secretions of the pancreas and intestines; protects the arteries; has antioxidant qualities; reduces cholesterol. It is an excellent cholagogue (increases the flow of bile to the duodenum). Helps for all hepatic disorders. It is recommendable to take one spoonful of oil in a glass of warm water during fasting. External use: Tones and smoothes the skin and hair, giving them a shiny look. Leaves made into a tea alleviate high blood pressure, and renal or arteriosclerosis problems. Leaves and bark made into a tea or cooked reduce fever and alleviate neuralgia.

**Chard.** Rich in vitamin A, B, folic acid and iron.

**Therapeutic Indication**: Useful in counteracting inflammation of the kidneys and for retention of liquids. Helps the gallbladder. Relieves constipation and acts as a digestive tonic. External use: leaves may be used as a poultice for acne and all types of abscesses and burns.

**Avocado**. The avocado is eaten ripe and it has a high nutritive and energetic value, as it has nearly all the calories of a dietary meal. It has more than twelve minerals: sodium, phosphorous, potassium, magnesium, iron, calcium, copper, sulfur, chloride, manganese, etc. It has eleven vitamins: C, K, B1, B2, B3, B5, B6 and B9. Its high levels of oil contain pro-vitamins A, D and E. It contains proteins, fats and carbohydrates in sufficient proportion for you to eat one every day.

**Therapeutic Indication**: Invigorates the brain and the optic nerve. It is energetic, dilates blood vessels, reduces cholesterol, is rich in glutathione and is a powerful antioxidant. Recommended as an ideal for children. Recommendable for overwork and weakness. External use: protects and softens the skin, ideal for sensitive skin.

**Garlic**. Its intensive use dates back many centuries. The unusual odor of garlic is produced by a very volatile essential oil, nearly all of which is made up of allyl sulfur. It was considered as sacred in olden days. It contains vitamins C, B1, B3, and pro-vitamin A, and the minerals iron, magnesium, sodium, calcium potassium and phosphorous: It also has proteins, cellulose, fat, carbohydrates, water, ash, omega 3 and other elements.

**Therapeutic Indication**: Garlic may be used to help all body systems. It purifies, is a natural antibiotic, and it invigorates, stimulates and vitalizes the organism. It is an appetizer; improves bacteria and helps intestinal flora. It reduces cholesterol, balances blood pressure, invigorates the heart, and dissolves mucus in the cavities of the frontal and maxillary sinuses, the lungs and bronchi. It may be used as a cough medicine. People who snore should eat one clove of garlic four times a day. Helps tuberculosis, and powerful against parasites. To expel intestinal worms, take 25 grams of garlic a day in a glass of milk or water that has been boiled for twenty minutes. Reduces poisons substances through sweating; increases the production of semen and stimulates the sexual function. It is diuretic and has anti-cancerous agents. The combination of onion, garlic and ginger is very healthy. It is recommendable to eat one or two cloves of garlic a day to keep healthy. One cup of light tea made from garlic, lemon balm or angelica drunk after each meal helps digestion, fermentation and alleviates intestinal gas. If bitten by an insect or stung by a bee, remove the stinger and rub the wound with garlic. Small cists and warts may be rubbed with garlic several times a day and they will disappear.

Chew a stalk of parsley, a few grains of anis, an apple or cumin in order to prevent strong-smelling breath. Kyolic non-artificially deodorized garlic tablets are recommended. Two counter-indications: Women breastfeeding their children are not recommended to eat garlic, nor people who have a skin infection or eczema.

**Artichoke**. Has a 50% content of potassium, high in calcium and other minerals, such as sodium, iron, magnesium, sulfur, copper, fluor, phosphorous, chloride and iodine. Vitamins include C, B1, B2 and B3, and proteins, carbohydrates and calories.

**Therapeutic Indication**: Recognized for its ability to detoxify and purify the blood. Reduces cholesterol. Its oils are useful for the metabolism and have a powerful stabilizing effect. Stimulates the function of intestine. Alleviates constipation, rheumatism, arthritis and diabetes. The nervous system stabilizes after eating artichoke for several weeks. Great help in hepatic disorders. Stimulates the production of bile and eliminates liquids. As a diuretic: squeeze 0.60 grams of leaves and add a bottle of white wine and pulp juice. Macerate for a week and strain. Drink one cup a day.

**Alfalfa**. The name of this wonderful herb means "the father of food". It has a high number of well balanced nutrients. Vitamins: C, pro-vitamin A, B1, B2, B5, B6, B9, and K; minerals: calcium, phosphorous, potassium, magnesium, sodium, chloride, sulfur, silicone and trace elements; eight essential amino acids; very rich in chlorophyll.

**Therapeutic Indication**: Chlorophyll is of great use for all the organism's systems. It vitalizes and prevents and combats infections. Chlorophyll and blood molecules are chemically similar, except that the main atom of chlorophyll is magnesium and the main atom of human blood is iron.

**Seaweed**. A sea vegetable that has existed since life on earth began and there are thousands of sweet water and saltwater species. It has a high content of proteins, salts, minerals, trace elements and vitamins A, C and D, and some complex B, particularly B12. **Kelp** is very valuable. It helps to build the organism and is rich in iron, minerals, vitamins, trace elements and other vital components.

**Spirulina seaweed** is dark green, has a high content of beta carotene, other carotenoids and phytonutrients; 64% of protein, essential and non-essential amino acids, vitamins, such as complex B, among other minerals such as iron, fatty acids, chlorophyll, RNA, DNA. **Hijiki seaweed** is rich in minerals, basically potassium, iron and calcium and oleaginous elements, and vitamin B12. **Wakame seaweed** is rich in calcium, potassium and vitamins of group B and C. **Nori seaweed** is rich in protein, phosphorous and pro-vitamin A.

**Therapeutic Indication**: An excellent source of energy. Use for afflictions related to lack of iodine, and against goiter and scurvy. Acts as a protecting agent against mucus. People with acne should not eat much seaweed. The action of **parda seaweed** is antibacterial and antiviral. **Nori seaweed** kills bacteria and is useful for healing ulcers. **Spirulina seaweed** is an essential part of children's diet due to its high nutritional content. Eat half an hour before any meal in order to reduce your appetite. It is highly important for vegetarian people.

**Amaranth**. It was an important food from pre-Hispanic Mexico. For the last one hundred years it has been essential in China, Tibet, Nepal, India and Pakistan. It has high-quality proteins much more than other cereals. Vitamins: B1, B2, B3, A, C, and complex B. Its seeds contain the minerals: potassium, sodium, magnesium, copper, manganese, nickel, iron, calcium and zinc. It is rich in lipids, amino acids, ash, raw fiber and lysine.

**Therapeutic Indication**: Regulates insulin due to its zinc content. Of high nutritive value and supports the organism as a whole.

**Celery**. It is a shame that celery is not to the taste of all palates. It has an excellent balance of nutritional elements. It has a high content of organic sodium, potassium, calcium, iron, manganese, magnesium, phosphorous, chloride, copper, sulfur and zinc. Vitamins: C, E, B1, B2, B3, B5, B6, B9, H. Proteins and carbohydrates. Quickly recovers all nutriments lost through sweating.

**Therapeutic Indication**: An excellent appetizer. Calms the nervous system; acts as a general tonic and anti-acidic. Purifying and eliminates the toxicity of cancerous agents, such as cigarette smoke. Regulates the pH of the blood and blood pressure. Useful for problems of the liver, the gallbladder, menstruation and spleen. It is diuretic and alleviates gallstones, constipation, arthritis and rheum. Excellent for diabetics. Relieves headache, ovaries, prostate glands and genital glands. Leaves cooked in milk relieve asthma, pulmonary catarrh and clear the voice.

**Beetroot**. Should be eaten raw, so as to make the most of its aminoacids and minerals that include: iron, sodium, potassium, sulfur, phosphorous, calcium, chloride, magnesium, manganese, copper, zinc, and asparagines. It is high in folic acid (B9). Vitamins: A, C, B1, B2, B3, B5, B6. High in assimilable carbohydrates. Carbohydrates increase when cooked and are concentrated without loosing their mineral content, although other vitamins are reduced.

**Therapeutic Indication**: Excellent as a rebuilder during convalescence (combined with carrot and cucumber juice); excellent for rebuilding the cells and blood cells (anti-anemic); detoxifies the liver, and cleans the spleen, kidneys and prostate gland; regulates pH in the digestive system; controls peristaltic movement and strengthens the assimilation of food; helps reproductive and cerebral functions and the normal metabolism of glucose and the bone structure; useful during menopause, menstruation and sexual weakness. Not recommended for diabetics due to its high sugar content, but is recommendable for young people and people who enjoy sports. Due to its content of oxalates and uric acid , it is not recommendable for people who have renal stones or high levels of uric acid.

**Broccoli**. A variety of cabbage. Has many more nutritional qualities than cauliflower and Brussels sprouts; contains a high quantity of beta carotene, vitamin C, B2, indoles and chlorophyll that makes it more digestible. A cup of steamed broccoli gives you all the vitamin A you need, twice the vitamin C, 6% of vitamin B3, 9% of calcium, 12% of phosphorous, 10% of iron, 20% of dietetic fiber, 5 grams of protein, 45 calories, potassium and folic acid.

**Therapeutic Indication**: Has an excellent antioxidant action. Invigorates the digestive system, protects the intestine, relieves constipation and prevents hemorrhoids. Purifies. It is diuretic and laxative; reduces the risk of cancer, particularly lung cancer, cancer of the colon (carbon indole 3 emulsifies estrogen in women, reducing the possibility of breast cancer); prevents ulcers and combats viruses. May it cause stomach problems? Yes, due to its high content of sulfur and grade of fermentation. Cook broccoli in boiling water with a pinch of baking soda.

**Pumpkin.** Contains proteins, calories, minerals: potassium, sodium, sulfur, chloride, calcium, phosphorous, iron and copper, and vitamins C, B1, B2, B3 and pro-vitamin A in major quantities.

**Therapeutic Indication:** A light stimulant for kidneys. Pips are used to expel tapeworms from the intestines.

**Onions.** Many centuries ago, the Egyptians believed the onion plant to be sacred as it was a genuine pharmaceutical product and appears painted on tombs. It has a strong flavor and has much to do with the construction of our organism, being more effective when eaten raw. Contains vitamins A, C, E, B1, B2, B3, B5, B6, B9, K, P, minerals, salts, sugars and starch.

**Therapeutic Indication:** An excellent stimulant for the nervous system (it has an excellent calming effect), the hepatic system and the renal system. Diuretic, a stimulant, anti-scorbutic and is also an aphrodisiac. Helps the respiratory system; eliminates mucus and purifies the humors of the organism; stimulates bacteria that benefit the intestine and combat constipation; purifies blood and stimulates the production of blood; neutralizes excess cholesterol; prevents coagulation in arteriosclerosis; eliminates abscess and ulcers; useful for rheum and deforming arthritis and for problems of the spleen and cystitis. Its curative value increases when taken with garlic and ginger. Raw sliced onion and turnip is useful for tumors and kidney stones when taken daily. People with ulcers, colitis or high blood pressure should not eat too much.

**External use**: Crushed onion juice helps growth of hair and invigorates it. Onion soup is good for the nerves. Onion soaked in vinegar for two hours may be applied to varicose veins and reduces skin blotches; apply raw on the skin in the diseased area. Eliminates worms when boiled with milk. In the form of a poultice it cures migraine and relieves rheumatism. The fine film between layers is an excellent antiseptic for wounds, ulcers, sores, etc. Soak a piece of cotton wool with onion juice and place on the hole left by tooth decay; it relieves neuralgia.

**Cabbage** There is a variety of cabbage, such as white, purple and green. When eaten raw it aids digestion, but when mixed, it causes flatulence. It is recommendable to eat it as a broth by which it retains must of its qualities. It contains proteins, carbohydrates, calories, phenols and indoles, which have protective qualities, plus vitamins A, C, B1, B2, B3, B5, B6, B9, H and U; minerals: potassium, sodium, calcium, silica, chloride, manganese, phosphorous, iron, magnesium, copper and zinc. It has a high content of organic sulfur.

**Red cabbage.** Rich in vitamin C, folic acid, potassium, phosphorous, magnesium, fibers and phito-chemical substances that provide protection against cancer. It contains flavonoids such as antonianos whose cyanidin gives the cabbage its purple color, and quercitine that is an anti-inflammatory and anti-cancerigenic.

**Therapeutic Indication:** Its antioxidants help prevent cancer of the colon and breast cancer. Vitamin U cures gastric or duodenal ulcers. Stimulates the immune system; useful for intestinal constipation; has purification properties; prevents arthritis and inflammation; eliminates intestinal worms; purifies the organism; regularizes the function of the stomach, the intestine and the liver, and attenuates gastric pain; balances the nervous system; helps the heart; helps regeneration of the cells; keeps the skin and hair healthy; increases the potency of men. **External use:** its leaves refresh the skin and may be applied as a poultice on swellings areas, wounds and difficult cases of rheumatism.

**Brussels sprouts.** Its nutritional qualities are similar to those of broccoli, but to a lesser extent. Contains proteins, carbohydrates, calories, indoles and fenoles. Provides all vitamin C (twice as much as oranges) if eaten raw. Vitamins: B1, B2, B3, B5, B6, B9 and H; minerals: sulfur, potassium, phosphorous, chloride, calcium, iron, sodium magnesium, manganese, copper and zinc. Should be cooked whole so that they do not loose their mineral salts.

**Therapeutic Indication:** Diuretic. Has therapeutic qualities similar to those of broccoli and cauliflower. Brussels sprout and green bean juice is excellent for diabetic adults.

**Horsetail.** Has a large quantity of silica and when you look at its leaves under a magnifying glass, you can see small, brilliant fragments. It is notable for replenishing minerals, more so than calcium.

**Therapeutic Indication:** Helps to join fractured bones and helps prevent rickets; useful for urinary incontinence and urine with blood. Boil in a liter of water for half an hour and drink between meals at room temperature.

**Cauliflower.** A compact, fleshy and soft flower. Contains proteins, carbohydrates, fats, cellulose and water; minerals: calcium, iron, chloride, phosphorous, potassium, sodium, magnesium and zinc and a high quantity of vitamins A, C, B1, B2, K, PP, B9 (folic acid) and a little vitamin E, and beta carotene.

**Therapeutic Indication:** Excellent for alkalinizing the organism; purifies and is anti-anemic; useful for problems of the liver and kidneys; useful in treating arthritis, gout and rheumatism;

stimulates the organism's defensive systems; helps to cure gastritis and ulcers. Diuretic, laxative and purifying. Do not throw cooking water away; use it for soups and stews.

**Peas.** Contain sufficient nutritional elements; rich in vitamin C, folic acid and complex B. Also contain iron, phosphorous, carbohydrates, fiber and are an excellent source of natural protein. Preferably eat uncooked.

**Therapeutic Indication:** Digestive and relieve constipation; reconstitute and replenish minerals; anti-cancerigenic; reduces levels of cholesterol; helps the liver. According to tradition, they are famous for their anti-fertility properties. People with liver and renal problems and arteriosclerosis should avoid eating them dry, as they are not easily digestible and may cause flatulence.

**Dandelion.** Contains very high levels of potassium, sodium and calcium, iron, magnesium and phosphorous, manganese, folic acid (B9), silica and bioflavonoids. High in vitamins A, C, B1, B2.

**Therapeutic Indication:** Strengthens the bones, spinal column and teeth (best taken with carrot juice and turnip leaves). A powerful cleaning and detoxifying agent for the liver, gallbladder and nervous system, if sugar and starch are eliminated from the diet; a great purifier of blood and has anti-anemic properties; removes kidney stones and gallstones; it is diuretic; cleans and protects the skin; cures asthma; makes warts disappear and strengthens nails and hair. Drink as a tea after meals to treat acidity in the stomach. Dry leaves, toasted and ground have a beneficial effect on digestion and rheum. You can toast the roots and use them to make a coffee substitute or mix with coffee. External use: the leaves and roots are used as tincture to treat psoriasis, eczema and acne.

**Green beans.** Contain proteins, carbohydrates, calories, vitamins A, C, B1, B2, B3, B5 and B6 and the minerals sodium, potassium, calcium, phosphorous, chloride, magnesium, manganese, iron, copper and zinc.

**Therapeutic Indication:** Stimulates the nervous system; useful for gout and convalescence; may stimulate the production of insulin if combined with Brussels sprouts. Drink a glass of juice a day.

**Asparagus.** A very much appreciated vegetable. Light in calories, contains fiber and essential and powerful oils; vitamins: B1, B2, B3, B5, B6, B9 and H; minerals: potassium, sulfur, phosphorous, calcium, sodium, iron, chloride, copper, magnesium, manganese and zinc.

**Therapeutic Indication:** Invigorates the nervous system; purifies the blood; regulates glandular and digestive problems; improves circulation; dissolves the crystals of inorganic oxalic acid in the kidneys produced by to the asparagine alkaloid that it contains. It is diuretic, and may be used in moderate cases of cystitis or prostatis. May be used as a light laxative; useful for hydropsy and inflammation of the spleen. People who suffer from renal inflammation or who have diabetes or gout should eat small quantities under strict medical supervision. The crushed seeds mixed with honey or sugar in equal parts eases persisting vomiting and reduces inflammation of the liver. Eat from the tip of a spoon.

**Spinach.** We owe spinach to the Arabs. For the digestive tract it is the best and most vital source type of food. It has a sufficient quantity of oxalic acid, an element that together with calcium maintains and stimulates the peristaltic movement of the intestine. When cooked, it turns into an inorganic element (crystals that deposit themselves in the kidneys) and when eaten together with calcium, both destroy them. Contains highly concentrated minerals, vitamins, proteins, and calories. Minerals: calcium, sodium, potassium, magnesium, phosphorous, sulfur, chloride, iron and copper; vitamins: A, C, B1, B2, B3, B5, B9 and H.

**Therapeutic Indication:** Purifies, rebuilds and regenerates the digestive tract; regulates the functioning of the intestines; relieves constipation. It is recommendable not to eat much spinach to ease inflammation of the digestive system. Increases red blood cells; purifies, regenerates and revitalizes blood. It is a cardiac invigorator; it stimulates the liver, the lymphatic gland and the pancreatic function; contains antioxidants; has reconstituting properties; provides protection against cancer; acts a a laxative; supports the nervous system. Fiber helps to decrease cholesterol. Its content in uric and oxalic acid makes it recommendable to be eaten in small quantities by people who suffer from gout, renal stones or arthritis. When cooked, spinach should be kept for no longer than 24 hours, as its toxic substances increase immediately; the same happens if it is tinned or frozen.

**Jamaica.** Contains vitamin C and complex B.

**Therapeutic Indication:** An excellent diuretic; useful for treating kidney stones, constipation, dysentery, fever, inflammation of the gums, loosing weight and reducing defenses of the organism; reduces triglycerides and cholesterol. Boil the flower in water and strain. Drink as water once a day. Calyxes are used as colorants for certain types of food.

**Fennel.** The Egyptians, Greeks and Romans included fennel as part of their diet. It is part of the celery family and has similar nutritional values. It contains stimulating properties, a large quantity of essential oils, carbohydrates, fats, calories, potassium, calcium, iron, and phosphorous, vitamins A, complex B and a very high content of vitamin C.

**Therapeutic Indication:** Helps during convalescence and migraine; useful for stomach indigestion when mixed with apple juice; eliminates intestinal gas; increases red blood cells. Best when mixed with carrot and beetroot. Diuretic. Take with carrot juice for the eyesight.

**Mushrooms.** There are many varieties, some of which are highly toxic. It is best to buy them in specialized shops. They are high in potassium, manganese, copper, selenium, iodine and zinc. They replace meat as a source of protein.

**Therapeutic Indication:** The Chinese and Japanese consider mushrooms as a source of longevity. They strengthen the organism's defenses, prevent cancer and reduce cholesterol, relieve headaches and act as a stimulant, they thin the blood and prevent heart attacks.

**Ginger.** A root that contains a glucoside called gingerol, volatile oil, gum starch, sugar and fatty material. Is an excellent food and in general appetizing, stimulating and good for the stomach. Together with garlic and onion it increases nutritional value.

**Therapeutic Indication:** Stimulates and nourishes the nervous system and cerebral function; provides men vitality; removes toxins from the body; stimulates digestion; cleans the kidneys and intestines; useful for bronchitis, colds, sore throat, cough, constipation, diarrhea, circulation, colic and dyspepsia; eases menstrual pain; relieves menstrual colic and general fatigue. In a syrup combined with red pepper it helps to decongest the nasal cavities.

**Lettuce.** The greener the leaves the better. Contains alkaloids that have a powerful effect, vitamins A, C, E, B1, B2, B3, B5, B6, B9; and minerals: potassium, iodine, phosphorous, iron, magnesium, calcium, cobalt, sulfur, copper chloride, arsenic and zinc.

**Therapeutic Indication:** Has a sedative effect and is excellent for insomnia, better taken not cooked. It is a tonic for the nervous system, glands and digestive organs; constipation; detoxifies the organism; combats stomach acidity; mineralizes the blood; it is diuretic and laxative. Fertility. The root and the trunk when cooked help stomach ache, irritation and constipation.

**Lime.** Has a high quantity of malic, acidic, formic, and citric acids, and vitamin C and, in lesser quantities, vitamins B1, B6, B3 and B5; minerals: potassium, calcium, iron, phosphorous, magnesium, sodium and essential oil that refreshes the organism. It used to be considered as more of a medicine than a fruit. It has nutritional and medicinal qualities that helps prevent and cure many afflictions at all ages. The lime tree provides everything: the juice of the fruit, peel, pips, leaves, flowers, bark and roots.

**Therapeutic Indication:** Lime juice is physiological water with antiseptic and detoxifying properties and high nutritional value that makes it a very effective cure for fever, rheum, gout, arthritis, inflammation of the liver and the gallbladder and for malaria and syphilis. Purifies the blood; acts a general tonic; useful for regenerating the cells; it is astringent and diuretic; lime juice with hot water taken before breakfast cleans mucus in the throat and the stomach and helps to break the fast. It is recommended drink warm lime juice after eating much. If you want to loose weight, drink lime juice for 20 days, twice a day: first day one lime, second day two limes, third day three limes, etc. until reaching the tenth day when you use the reverse method and decrease your lime intake until the end of the cure. **Lime pips** are excellent for in removing all types of worms. Mix with honey and take a spoonful before breakfast, the effect of which lasts between 4-5 days. **Leaves** in tea help digestion. Before breakfast it activates secretion of gastric juices. The **Azahar flower** is a sedative of the nervous system; take three times a day. The **root** may be used to ease problems of the liver and the gallbladder. Cook 40 grams per liter of water and drink three cups a day. **Bark** provides essential oil that refreshes the organism. May be applied externally to treat sunburn and insect bites. Dice and macerate the **peel** in warm water for twelve hours and take for depression, migraine, catarrh and the skin.

**Turnip**. A root vegetable low in nutrients; eat cooked and in small quantities. Contains proteins, carbohydrates, calories and vitamins A, C, E, H, B1, B2, B3, B5, B6 and B9; and minerals: sodium, chloride, iron, sulfur, copper and magnesium. Raw leaves are a concentrated source of calcium, potassium and vitamins.

**Therapeutic Indication**: Of great help to the nervous and muscular system. Slightly expectorant. Juice with sugar not only tastes nice, but also calms pulmonary irritations and hacking coughs; regulates cholesterol; useful for high pressure, rheum and hemorrhoids; helps the kidneys; has great fortifying properties.

**Cactus (Nopal).** There are many species and is also known as "green gold". It can be found over the entire American continent and is part of the cactus family. It is a wild plant that grows in cold and desert regions and has an edible fruit called prickly pear. The Aztecs called it the "plant of life" because it never dies. When it dries it produces another plant. It is a major source of soluble and insoluble digestive fiber: lignin, cellulose, hemi-cellulose, pectin and mucilage that, together with the 17 amino acids, help to remove toxins. Contains large quantities of vitamins: A, C, B2, B6, and K; minerals: a high proportion of calcium, magnesium, sodium, potassium, iron and copper. Contain seventeen amino acids, both essential and non-essential, carbohydrates and acts as a natural antibiotic.

**Therapeutic Indication:** The soluble fiber creates a sensation of satiation and decreases hunger and aids digestion. It may relieve and prevent constipation, hemorrhoids and prevent cancer of the colon. The presence of soluble fiber in the digestive tube delays absorption of nutrients and makes them pass more slowly into the blood, thus facilitating their elimination. Protects gastrointestinal mucus; helps to prevent, reduce and control the levels of glucose in the blood, therefore it is of incalculable value for people with diabetes. Reduces cholesterol and triglycerides. When grilled it helps the liver, inflammation of the bladder, eases bronchial afflictions of and reduces cystitis irritation. External use: May be used for healing. Grill the fleshy part on one side and apply as a poultice on spots, inflammations, and boils. Note: if you do not like the sap, you may buy it dehydrated.

**Potatoes.** There are many varieties. May be kept for years in the same ground in which they grow, thus increasing their starch content. Contain one third of vitamin C of the daily consumption that the organism needs. It is a major source of potassium, phosphorous, chloride, sulfur, magnesium, calcium, iron, sodium, and copper; vitamins: H, K, PP, B1, B2, B3, B5, B6, B9, and complex B. Contains starch, cellulose, ash, albumin, fat and water. Contains penicillin, in a greater proportion if dehydrated. Red potatoes contain antioxidants that prevent deterioration of the cells (as do sweet potatoes and red corn). The skin is alkaline and balances acidity of the pulp, therefore it should preferably be eaten raw. Remove the buds and green parts because they contain solanine, a toxic alkaloid.

**Therapeutic Indication:** Before breakfast, raw potato removes uric acid. A broth made from the skin softens the articulations that have been hardened by arthritis or rheum. Potato, celery and carrot juice is excellent for gastric and duodenal ulcers, hemorrhoids, constipation, and pulmonary emphysema and invigorates the nervous and muscular system. Potassium helps to prevent cerebral-vascular problems and hypertension. White potato contains protease inhibitors that act against cancer. Grill potato helps to control sugar levels. "You should not eat potatoes when there is a venereal disease or aphrodisiac trends", says Dr. Norman W. Walter. External use: apply to the skin for infections and blotches. When used as a poultice it to relieve inflammation.

**Cucumber.** Contains high quantities of potassium and mineral salts: calcium, phosphorous, chloride, sodium, magnesium, manganese, sulfur, silica, iron, copper, zinc, iodine and sulfur; average content of vitamins: C, B1, B2, B3, B5, B6, B9; large quantity of biological water.

**Therapeutic Indication:** Has purifying and revitalizing properties; stimulates the nervous system; invigorates and strengthens the heart and muscles; provides the skin cells elasticity; helps growth of nails and hair; useful for problems of high pressure, arthritis, rheum, goat; best when combined with spinach, carrot, and lettuce juice. Useful for treating ulcerous colitis. It is diuretic and sooths inflammation; eliminates uric acid; relieves constipation. External use: Leaves the skin smooth. Excellent healing properties. Conserve the juice by boiling it for one minute: two parts of juice for one of alcohol.

**Parsley.** Contains a high quantity of vitamin C and provitamin A and B1, B2, B3, B5, B6, B9 and H; it has a high content of iron, calcium and magnesium, in addition to potassium, chloride, phosphorous and copper. Proteins and calories. Oligoelements. Contains a high concentration of antioxidants. Freeze the leaves.

**Therapeutic Indication:** General stimulant of the organism; oxygenates the blood; essential for oxygenating the metabolism and maintaining the normal function of the suprarenal and thyroid glands; reconstitutes the blood; increases red blood cells; cleans the liver, kidneys and urinary tract; regulates calcium. It is a nervous and muscular relaxant; it has excellent anti-cancerigenic properties; excellent for the sight and capillary system. Chew when birth pain begins and to improve breath. "It is one of the best diuretics for curing hydropsy", says Father Kniepp. External use: Apply to bee stings, insect bites or slight burns.

**Pepper.** There is an enormous variety in size, taste and color, such as red, green, yellow, brown, sweet, etc. Paprika may be obtained by grinding dry peppers. Contains high concentration of vitamin C that is an antioxidant, complex B, beta-carotene, minerals: calcium, phosphorous, iron, copper, potassium, sodium, zinc, water, glucides, lipids, proteins, and fiber. Contains a high quantity of silica that is good for the hair and nails.

**Therapeutic use:** Eases diarrhea, colic, flatulence and gas; has excellent anti-inflammation properties and acts as a bactericide, stimulant, tonic and appetizer. Stimulates the secretion of saliva and gastric uses and helps peristalsis of the intestine. Excellent for influenza, bronchitis, asthma, and respiratory infections. Supports the circulatory system and regulates blood pressure.

Useful for arteriosclerosis, cancer, and cataracts. Taking it with carrot and spinach juices helps you to relax. It is slow to digest, is normally due to not chewing it well enough.

**Leek.** See garlic. Applicable to leek.

**Radish.** Due to its strong flavor it is preferable to combine it with other vegetables to reduce its strong taste. Use the roots and leaves. Has a high content of iodine, potassium, sodium and other mineral salts, such as iron, magnesium, sulfur, calcium, phosphorous, manganese and chloride. Vitamins C and B1. Protectors: indoles and fenoles

**Therapeutic Indication:** Excellent for the respiratory system; dissolves all the body's mucus, mainly in the nose and maxillary and frontal sinuses, while at the same time helping to regenerate membranes. The juice combined with carrot juice is excellent for restoring the mucus membranes of the entire body. The roots and leaves have purifying qualities and combat cold and catarrh. The hot radish is more powerful and has the same applications.

**Red tomato.** Tomato originates from the word "tomatl" as the Mexicans call it. When fresh and raw it has an alkaline reaction. Its vital and balanced elements mineralize the blood. It has 50% more vitamin C than that recommended for daily intake. It is high in potassium, calcium, sodium, magnesium and contains other minerals such as sulfur, manganese, iron, chloride, fluorine, phosphorous, copper, cobalt and zinc. Vitamins: A, D, E, K, P, B1, B2, B3, B5, B6, B9. It is low in calories and sugars, has some oxalic acid and a high content of citric and malic acid necessary for metabolism of food. It is best not to combine it with fruit.

**Therapeutic Indication:** It generally invigorates the whole body, particularly the liver and the pancreas. It has purifying qualities; it is an excellent diuretic, and mineralizes and alkalinizes the organism. It contains an antioxidant called licopene, an anticancerous compound. It prevents cancer of the pancreas and uterine neck; prevents scurvy, bleeding gums and muscular fatigue. It is involved in transmitting nervous impulses and muscular concentration. Helps in digestion and constipation; useful for bronchial problems, hypertension, arthritis, gouts and rheum; may be used to treat anemia (together with carrots and spinach).

**Purslane.** An excellent source of nutrients, mineral salts and vitamins.

**Therapeutic Indication:** Helps to support the urinary system and remove gallstones from the bladder. Cooked leaves may be taken to reduce fever. Drink purslane juice before going to bed to get rid of insomnia.

**Carrots.** Very important for the human diet as raw carrots constitute a major source of minerals, vitamins, sugars and carotenes. Carrot juice is one of the most versatile, healthy and delicious there is. Its orange color is due to its high content of beta-carotene. Contains minerals: sodium, potassium, phosphorous, calcium, magnesium, chloride, sulfur, iron, manganese and copper; vitamins of the group B, C, D, E, G, K, H and provides much vitamin A.

**Therapeutic Indication**: It is alkaline, antioxidant, purifies the blood and strengthens the immune system. Protects the arteries and invigorates the intestinal walls. Excellent for all systems of the body as it disinfects repairs, invigorates and strengthens them. Useful for the skin, teeth, colon, ulcers, sight, nerves, sinusitis and cancer. Juice taken before breakfast is anthelmintic, increases visual acuteness, night vision and heals afflictions of the liver. Juice combined with beetroot and coconut cleans the kidneys and the gallbladder. External use: whole fresh leaves applied on burns, shredded on ulcers and purulent wounds that are difficult to heal.

**Eggplant**. First originated in India, later Arabs took it to Europe. It is poor as a source of nutrition. It contains less vitamins and minerals than any other vegetable. Vitamins: A, B, C; minerals: cooper, magnesium, calcium, potassium, phosphorous, zinc, and bioflavonoids. It has a fleshy pulp that can be eaten grilled, breaded, baked, in puree, etcetera.

**Therapeutic indication**: Its best use is as laxative due to the cellulose it contains. Reduces cholesterol. Relaxes the nervous system. Stimulates the liver and pancreas function. Counter indicated in heart diseases due to the solanine substance it contains. External use: the leaves are used as poultice in inflammation, relieve skin problems including burnings. It is recommended to include it for losing weight. When the eggplant is green (not ripe), it is highly toxic and raw it is indigested.

Watercress. It has a strong flavor. It contains one of the best sources of iodine and other minerals such as: sulfur, phosphorous, potassium, sodium, iron, calcium, and chloride. Vitamins it contains: pro-vitamin A, B1, B2, B5, H, and PP.

**Therapeutic indication**: Excellent body cleanser. Revitalizing and refreshing. It cleans the digestive system, the liver and the gallbladder. Good for tuberculosis treatment, high blood pressure and diabetes. It is one of the best stimulants and expectorants. Helps prevent some types of cancer. Moderate use is recommended and when mixing it with other vegetables. Cultivated watercress is recommended instead of the wild one, since the latter may contain a parasitic worm transmitted by animal wastes. It is eaten in salads containing minerals. In 80g dose of watercress juice, administered in equal parts through the day, it helps as diuretic and anti-scorbutic. Capes are watercress buds.

**Vegetable soup**

Boil the amount of water you wish and then add unpeeled vegetables: carrot, turnip, chayote, cauliflowers stalks, broccoli stalks, celery stalks with their leaves, all leaves that you have handy, and onion, garlic, leek, etc. Boil for two hours. Strain and throw the vegetables away as they have no nutritional value. Use the broth for preparing soups and stews.

# 3. Whole grain

**Whole grain** is, in essence, the presence and power of the miracle of our existence. It has a wealth of proteins, minerals and vitamins. Whole grain includes cereals, legumes, oleaginous products, seeds, fruit and raw vegetables. It contains the 12 minerals: sulfur, calcium, fluoride, fluorine, phosphorous, silica, sodium, potassium, iron, magnesium, iodine, manganese, selenium, carbon, hydrogen, nitrogen and oxygen. Natural foods contain flours and sugars that may be assimilated into the human organism.

<u>Cereals</u> have the following origins: wheat from Western Europe; corn from America, rice from Asia, oatmeal and rye from the southern hemisphere, and millet from Africa, all of which have been eaten for thousands of years, thanks to their source of concentrated energy, adaptability and abundant production. Rice, corn, wheat, oats, barley, rye, millet, and sorghum grown on stalks. They contain 80% flour; germs rich in vitamin B, E and F, minerals, fats and proteins, the fatty part of which includes lecithin that keeps cholesterol in a liquid form. Untreated seeds contain large quantities of phosphorous, sodium, manganese, copper, zinc, cobalt, iron, calcium, magnesium and are eliminated during the refining process, as is the cereal fiber whose function is to prevent constipation and facilitates low absorption of food and digestive fermentation. Whole or germinated cereals are easy to digest.

<u>Legumes</u> grow virtually anywhere in the world and adapt to various conditions of climate and soil that they enrich as they are nitrogen fixers. Legumes are characterized due to their high content of protein, between 17% and 25%; mineral salts include calcium, iron and magnesium; vitamins of group B, abundant carbohydrates and a low fat content (lower than any other protean food) and a high content of fiber. Soy beans and lentils (very protean), chickpeas, broad beans, peas, alfalfa, tamarind seeds and all varieties of beans grow on vines.

**Therapeutic Indication:** Lentils may be used to treat cases of anemia and convalescence, but have counter indications due to their high protean content for afflictions such as gout, rheum, arteriosclerosis, artrosis, and for old people, as excess protein produces toxic substances that damage the organism when they accumulate. Due to their high caloric content they should be consumed in moderation by people who have a slow pace of life. Not recommended for obese people with diabetes and a weak digestive system. Soft broad beans may be used to prevent cholesterol fixing itself in the blood vessels and the adipose degeneration of the liver.

**Note: For intestines not used to consume legumes, they** may cause gas, so it is recommendable to eat only a little until the intestinal tract becomes accustomed. Soaking beans before cooking improves digestion. Add salt near the end of cooking as this helps to harden skin. Old legumes ferment more so is better to germinate them. Dry legumes may be kept in glass receptacles to keep them fresh. **Legumes** complement their essential amino acids with **cereals**, forming a complete protein, thus achieving a good balance. Most legumes are high in lysine. Cereals have few amino acids, although they have containing metionine, scarce in legumes. A balanced combination for any diet is **1/3 legumes to 2/3 cereal.**

<u>Soy beans</u>. Its botanic name is Glucine Max and is a member of the legumes family. The name soy comes from old Chinese: Sou. In modern times it is called Ta Tou, which means "great bean". It is considered as one of the five sacred grains: rice, wheat, millet, barley and soy. The protean level of soy is excellent. It is the best known grain for substituting the protein of meat. It contains

essential amino acids, fatty acids and vitamins A, C, D, E, K, B1, B2, B3; and minerals: calcium, iron, phosphorous, sodium, magnesium and copper. The soy plant enriches the earth because it has a symbiotic relationship with the rhizobia bacteria that makes the earth more fertile and productive. The corn plant has a detrimental effect on the soil, so it may be sown alternately or together.

Soy is not only economic, but also very versatile. It can be used to make milk, yoghurt, tofu (cheese), okara, dough, germinates, texturized soy, coffee, flour, etc. Tofu contains 23% more calcium than cow's milk with alkaline composition. Okara contains proteins of very high nutritional value.

<u>**Soy milk**</u> (basic recipe)

1      cup of soy beans.
2 ½   liters of water
1      stick of cinnamon or vanilla
Brown sugar cone to taste.

Soak the beans between 12 and 16 hours (the water used for soaking is a good plant fertilizer). Wash well in order to avoid stomach upset. Boil half of the water and use the rest to crush the beans in the blender. Pour the mixture into the saucepan while the water is boiling and leave to simmer. Strain using a strainer covered with a cloth. Place the milk on the stove, and cinnamon and sugar and simmer for 15 to 20 minutes.

## Okara.

This is the part left over when juice is extracted from the beans. It contains proteins of high nutritional value. Okara contains essential fiber that helps the proper functioning of the intestine. It may be used to prepare a number of dishes: mincemeat, tortillas, bread, soup, etc. When making bread from corn flour or wheat, replaces one quarter of flour with Okara and it will be more nutritional. If Okara is well ground as dough (go) you may replace it with eggs and its bread will be more nutritional.

<u>**Tofu.**</u> (Cheese)

1   one cup of soaked soy beans
5 cups of water
 Two limes

Prepare the milk; it must be thin and warm. Add the lime little by little and stir it until well mixed. Let stand until set. Remove carefully and pour on a thin gauze (closed weave) and strain to remove the whey. Hold the corners of the cloth and submerge the curdle in cold water. When the cloth is dry it should come loose on its own. The dough remains white and smooth of cheese. If you wish, knead and add soy sauce or salt and condiment with garlic, onion, parsley, etc. and mould into the shape of cheese. Tofu whey should be transparent and have a sweet taste. If it is acid, you added too much lime or vinegar.

Note: in order to curdle soy milk, instead of lime you may use a spoonful of magnesium sulfate, sea salt or vinegar, or one spoonful of Worcestershire sauce dissolved in half a cup of water.

The whey is an excellent plant fertilizer. It may be used hot as soap for washing clothes, as a shampoo for the hair, as a skin cleansing lotion, to wash wooden floors and furniture, as well as broth for soups.

Tofu mayonnaise

1   cup of tofu
5   teaspoons of lime juice
5   teaspoons of oil
Salt and pepper to taste.
3   Cloves of crushed garlic or to taste.
Blend: add onion or parsley, diced colander or oregano or sesame seeds, etc., to taste.

**Therapeutic Indication**:   Proteins are involved in a wide range of vital processes, thousands of millions of cells of the muscles and of the organs that are constantly dying and renewing themselves. They help to build all the parts of the organism and to form the bones, muscles, tissues, the heart, blood, the balance of liquids, skin, hair and nails. The genistein that it contains prevents tumors. Tofu is recommended for problems of the circulatory system. Helps to produce estrogens and reduces cholesterol.

## Wheat

Wheat is produced around the world and there are a number of varieties. It is one of our most important basic foods. It is a gramineous plant of the cereal group. It has all the important elements for maintaining the human organism. Whole wheat is the most balanced type. It contains oxygen, carbon, nitrogen, hydrogen, calcium, chloride, sulfur, fluorine, iron, phosphorous, thiamine (B1), riboflavin (B2), folic acid (B3), pantenol (B5), vegetable oil, protein, white flour of little nutritional value and cellulose. Proteins, phosphates and nitrates help to form the six biochemical salts that make up the human organism. Whole grain contains lots of nutrients.

Wheat is divided into four parts: bran, the protein layer (gluten), starch and germ. Semola, germ, bran, wheat germ oil and flour are extracted from wheat.

**Refined flour** losses nearly all its nutrients and thus loses its qualities as a restorative and vitalizing food that improves health (it is eaten most in the form of white bread).

**Germ** is the embryo of the grain and the most nutritional part thanks to its major contribution of vitamin E, proteins, fat, etc.

**Bran** is the outer husk of wheat. It is made up of two vegetable fibers that are not degraded by the human digestive system. It is a residue food that increases in volume when absorbing water and the volume of the bolus and fecal bolus. It is the cellulose that acts as stimulant of peristaltic movement (contraction and expansion) of the intestine and contains a large quantity of vitamins and minerals. It is excellent for a slimming diet as it gives you a sensation of satiation without producing calories.

**Gluten** is the protein of wheat. Starch has been eliminated. It is a very versatile food, easy to prepare, and does not have any toxins, uric acid. It is always fresh, healthy and nutritional, as well as being economical.

**Preparation**: 2 kilos of whole meal flour or white flour. Add water as necessary.

**Method**: Place the flour in a recipient and add water gradually until it forms a smooth dough. Cover the dough with water in the recipient. Leave overnight or for six hours. Wash the dough as if it were kneading. The water turns white and is thrown away. Keep washing with clean water until it remains slightly white. Its volume reduces when the starch is removed, leaving only the protein. Cover once again with clean water and leave for 1 or 2 hours. Tip water away and roll the dough into small balls. You may then beat them to make into steaks, or cut it into small squares, strips or leave them whole; depending on the dish you wish to prepare (you will be able to prepare approximately 16 to 18 medium-sized steaks.). Some ten minutes before the two hours of soaking has finished, heat a saucepan of water and add herbs, garlic, onion, celery and any other herbs you have handy and season with sea salt or soy sauce. When the water comes to the boil, add gluten and leave to cook for 20 to 25 minutes; then remove from the stove and strain. They are now ready to be prepared as you wish: as meat any style, with green sauce, with mushrooms, etc.

**Germinated wheat** Whole wheat releases starch when it germinates and that is how its nutritional richness is assimilated to the maximum. It should be incorporated into your daily life, particularly for children who are growing up, for people with problems with anemia, decalcification and demineralization, those who suffer from fatigue, women who are pregnant or breast feeding, and old people (see germinates).

## Rice

Rice needs to be grown in wet lands. Whole rice is one of the basic elements of a macrobiotic and vegetarian diet. Rice is eaten all around the world and is the most important cereal after wheat, due to its high quantity of vitamins, minerals and oligoelements. It has a low content of fat, sodium and potassium. During the refining or bleaching process (when talc or glucose is added), rice looses nearly all its nutrients as these are found in the outer layer and in the germ.

Whole rice contains vitamin E and vitamins B2, B3 and complex B, calcium, iron, proteins, phosphorous, potassium and carbohydrates, and it is very high in cellulose that eases constipation.

Raw whole rice should be refrigerated. When whole rice is cooked with celery its nutritional value increases.

# Corn

There are many varieties of this gramineous plant that originated in America, although it is now grown throughout the world. Its nutritional value is similar to that of other cereals. It has a high content of carotenes –provitamin A- (that no other cereal has). It has a number of nutritional and energetic elements, including vitamins of the B group and minerals. Fifty-seven percent of its minerals salts are acid. Its cellulose content favors intestinal movement. Its high content of carbohydrates does not make it recommendable for obese people or people suffering from diabetes. Corn does not contain gluten, so its flour does not rise as wheat flour does. Corn, also called tender corn ("choclo" in Quechua) is collected when it is young. The **oil** obtained from corn germ is recommended for its high content of cholesterol in the blood.

There is a wide variety in Mexico and it may be used to prepare a number of delicious dishes, such as corn soup, enchiladas, tacos, chilaquiles, chalupas, panuchos, papadzules, totopos, pozole, gorditas, pastel de elote, biscuits , tamales, pinole, etc.1 Do you need a digestive? Drink atole made from corn and also use *cacahuazintle* corn and the grain of thick crushed corn for making Italian bread called "polenta".

1    Translator's note: All these dishes are particular to Mexico and corn
     is the basic ingredient used. Similar in style to the Indian chapatti.

# Barley

A gramineous plant similar to wheat, grown in many areas around the world, even as far north as the Artic Circle. It is resists changes in temperature and grows quickly in wet lands. It is an annual plant like rice. Barley has not been sufficiently appreciated although it is highly nutritional. It is rich in phosphorous, iron, magnesium and sodium. It is refreshing and easy to digest for delicate intestines. It is diuretic and helps in acute problems of the liver.

### Oats

Of the gramineous family. It is eaten around the world. It is an energetic food rich in mineral salts: fluorine, silica, sodium, carbohydrates and particularly phosphorous that is needed for the brain and nervous system. Unrefined oats remove the organism's useless acids. It is laxative, recommended for weak stomachs and is of great help for children's diet. Two spoonfuls of raw oatmeal mixed with fruit helps to reduce cholesterol.

### Rye

A long-stalk cereal similar to wheat and barley. Grown in poor soil and used for crop rotation. Very nutritional and high in organic salts and other nutritients.

# Germinates

The secret of life is encapsulated in all types of seeds. They all have the same basic structure. Life generates more life.

The germination process begins with seeds. First of all the seed absorbs water, its skin softens it and expands. It needs water until the embryo is released (this feeds of albumin) and keeps developing in the external environment. Once this process has taken place, it changes its nutritional content and changes from being an acidifying food of the blood to alkalinizing and it increases the nutritional value of proteins, vitamins, minerals, salts and carbohydrates.

**Enzymes** of seeds metabolize their proteins forming aminoacids that are easier to digest. Enzymes metabolize and transform and multiply all the nutrients of seeds, for example: the vitamins of the B complex increase by up to 1500%; vitamin C rivals citric acids, carbohydrates in malt sugar easy to digest providing abundant energy to the organism, etc.

When seeds germinate, they lose their starchy nature and at the last stage, when exposed to light, vitamin A and chlorophyll are formed. Chlorophyll is the best natural deodorant, a tonic for the blood and digestion and removes the effect of radiation that damages the organism.

**Germinates** are an easy food to prepare, complete and prodigious because they regenerate and rejuvenate. It is a fresh food, full of life and free of contamination, so as to nourish our organism. It may resolve the problem of food shortages around the world and may serve as a form of survival.

It may be eaten with salad, soup, sandwiches, hot meals, tacos, chop-suey, milkshakes, fruit juice, etc.

If you wish to give your body energy and health, think of germinates. They are excellent for the glandular system and the nervous system. **Germinates is the highest form of nutrients.** Wheat grass juice is a complete food and prevents the development of cancer. Its medical virtues are miraculous: it detoxifies the organism, purifies the blood, repairs the cells and nourishes the brain. It is sweet and at first it may cause nausea or dizziness, until the body gets used to it.

The seeds or grains are divided into two groups: hard and soft.

Soft beans and small seeds are of the soft group and they need to be soaked for two to four hours in four cups of water before being put out to germinate.

Small, large and dry seeds are of the hard grain group and they need to be soaked for between eighth to 10 ten in four cups of water before germinating. The water used for soaking may be used as a fertilizer for plants or may used to make soups.

- Small seeds: alfalfa, millet, sesame seed, clover, radish, mustard

- Seeds with husk: sunflower seeds, pumpkin, peanuts, almond, buck wheat.

- Small and dry seeds: wheat, rye, oats, barley.

- Soft beans: mungo beans and lentils.

- Large and dry beans: broad beans, pinto and canario beans

- Large and extra-dry grains: soy beans, chickpea, corn, dry peas.

**Note**: soy beans loose their power of germination one year after being harvested. In order to conserve seeds, keep them in a cool, dry place in metal, dark glass or plastic containers that are hermetically sealed to keep moisture out.

To keep germinates intact, refrigerate them for one week and dry them in an oven or in a frying pan on a low gas. Keep them whole or ground and they will last a long time. (keep them as grain).

You can add them to soups, salads, milkshakes, etc.

## Germination process

All you need is a warm place in your kitchen, a jar, a tray, a saucepan or a one-liter glass jar with a wide mouth, a few squares of cloth and some elastic bands. The process is the same as for all seeds, the only difference being soaking time and time of germination.

1. Wash seeds well and place them (after they have been soaked) in a wide-mouthed jar that has been well washed. There should be sufficient space for seeds to germinate.

2. Cover the mouth of the jar with a cloth and fixed with an elastic band to keep out garbage and insects.

3. Wash two or three times a day. There should only be damp, not soaked. They must be strained well so as not to give off a bad odor and so that they do not rot. The jar must be must be tipped face downwards and the seeds distributed evenly.

4. If it is hot, the germination process will speed up; if room temperature is low, it will take longer.

5. Jars should not be placed in direct sunlight.

6. The germination period ends when the shoot has reached its size, depending on the germinated seed.

7.  Old seeds that have shown no signs of shoots should be removed, otherwise they may rot the other shoots.

8.  When the germination period has ended and when the first leaves appear, it is recommendable to place the seed in strong sunlight for a few hours in order to increase chlorophyll content.

9.  Remove the husk from the seeds before eating.

## To germinate grain in large quantities:

1.  Use a hot punch to make a hole in a large plastic bucket. Add grain already soaked and leave them a space to germinate. Add water two or three times a day and place them in two bricks to drain the water. Cover with damp cloth and ensure that it remains so.

2.  Various types of seeds may germinate in a single receptacle, provided that they have the same germination time, for example: soft seeds with soft seeds.

3.  Some seeds do not germinate combined, for example, soy beans and all other hard beans and seeds with husk, such as sunflower seeds, pumpkin, etc.

4.  A delicious combination is alfalfa, mungo beans and lentils. Mix one third of each in the same jar. You may try your own mixtures!

| SEEDS | Germinating time (days) | Number of times to be watered a day | Harvest | Number of seeds | Production |
|---|---|---|---|---|---|
| Alfalfa | 3-6 | 2 | 3 cm. | 2 spoonfuls. | 3 cups |
| Almond | 3-5 | 3 | 1-2 cm. | ¼ cup | ¼ cup |
| Sesame seed | 3-4 | 3-5 | 2 cm. | ½ cup | 1 cup |
| Rice | 3-4 | 2-3 | 1-2 cm. | ½ cup | 1 ¼ cup |
| Oat | 3-4 | 1 | 2 cm. | 1 cup | 2 cups |
| Barley | 3-5 | 2-3 | 2 cm. | 1 cup | 3 cups |
| Rye | 3-4 | 2-3 | 2-3 cm. | ½ cup | 2 ¾ cups |
| Beans | 4-5 | 3 | 2-4 cm. | ½ cup | 2 cups |
| Mungo beans | 4-5 | 3-5 | 4 cm. | ½ cup | 2 ½ cups |
| Chickpeas | 4-5 | 4 | 1-2 cm. | 1 cup | 3 cups |

| | | | | | |
|---|---|---|---|---|---|
| Sunflower seeds | 4-5 | 2-3 | 3 cm. | 1 cup | 3 cups |
| Lentils | 3-4 | 2-3 | 2 cm. | 1 cup | 6 cups |
| Corn | 4-5 | 2-3 | 2 cm. | 1 cup | 2 cups |
| Soy | 4-5 | 5-6 | 4 cm. | ½ cup | 2 ½ cups |
| Wheat | 3-4 | 2-3 | 3 cm. | 1 cup | 3 ½ cups |

# 4. Oleaginous products

The most common oleaginous seeds or "dry fruits" are: almonds, sesame seeds, walnuts, pine nut, pistachio nuts, chestnuts, hazelnuts, amaranth, sunflower seeds, pumpkin seeds and Brazil nuts. Although peanuts belong to the leguminous family, they have nutrients that are very similar to those of the products in this group. They are all an excellent alternative to animal protein.

Over half the content of oleaginous products are lipids (fats) in which healthy unsaturated fatty acids, such as oleic acid (mainly found in walnuts and hazelnuts) and linoleic acid (abundant in nuts and peanuts) predominate, except for coconuts that contain saturated fat. Oleaginous products are rich in essential fatty acids and are vital in the formation of cellular membranes, particularly in nerve cells. They have a high quantity of phosphorous, magnesium, calcium, potassium, iron and oligoelements such as selenium and zinc (with antioxidating action). They do not have any vitamin C but are rich in B1 (thiamine), B2 (niacin) and folates and vitamin E. Vitamins B1 and E are destroyed during the toasting process. Almonds, sunflower seeds and peanuts have more than 20% of protein and considerable quantities of fiber that help intestinal movement and ease constipation. Moderate consumption is recommended. Nuts should be chewed well to avoid digestive problems. Pumpkin seeds and peanuts are very proteic, but of low quality due to their low content of lysine and metionine. They should be eaten with cereals and legumes. Almonds, nuts and Brazil nuts contain more protein per unit of weight than fresh eggs and are of excellent quality. Due to their high oil content they easily become stale so they should be conserved in hermetically sealed containers in the refrigerator. One hundred grams of oleaginous products provide 400 to 600 calories. Avoid fired and salted nuts.

**Almonds**. The almond is a typical Mediterranean tree. Sweet almond is the most healthy of the almonds, easy to digest and is completely assimilated. It has a considerable quantity of proteins. It is a good source of vitamins, minerals and predominates in healthy unsaturated fatty acids, oleic acid and linoleic acid. However, it is low in carbohydrates, which can be compensated by adding honey. It has a high quantity of oil that when extracted may be used externally and internally. Has 53% fat.

**Almond milk**: Blend seven to ten almonds with a glass of water and add a teaspoon of honey. May replace breast milk.

**Therapeutic Indication**:    Prevents cancer and helps the nervous system. Almond milk is healthy and refreshes the digestive system. If drunk before going to bed, it makes you sleepy and calms you down. Useful against anemia, malnutrition and diabetes. Almond oil (pure) reduces cholesterol and fat, and removes toxins and hunger; it keeps the skin healthy. Women should take two tablespoons before breakfast during menstruation. It acts as a very effective laxative. Total vegetarians use it for preparing mayonnaise without eggs.

**External use**:  May be applied to skin burns. The oil may be used to prepare creams that soften dry skin of the body, face, hands and feet.

**Sesame seeds**.  Although they are very small seeds, they constitute a very nutritional, complete, balanced and high-quality food. They contain proteins, fats, phosphates, lecithin and minerals, such as calcium, potassium and magnesium. Cold pressed oil is an excellent source of calcium. Raw sesame seeds are difficult to digest and when toasted they lose 60% of their nutritional value, therefore it its recommendable to crush them raw with a little water in order to make a butter, or mix them with flour to make tortillas or bread.

**Therapeutic Indication**:   An excellent tonic; an excellent and efficient regulator of the intestinal function due to its content of mucilage; increases physical and mental capacity; Helps the nervous system and of the brain; increases secretions of the pineal, pituitary and sexual glands; increases virility; reinforces the reproductive system. Women should take two tablespoons of raw oil before and after menstruation. External use: apply as a poultice to reduce fever.

**Hazelnuts.**  As with all oleaginous products, hazelnuts are a highly nutritional source of food, containing 54% fat.

**Therapeutic Indication:**   An excellent muscular tonic. Strengthens and invigorates sportsmen. They are astringent, thermal and excellent for chronic diarrhea.

**Peanuts.**   Peanuts have a very nutritional value. They contain proteins, carbohydrates, fat, vitamins B1, B2 and B3, and pro-vitamin A. Minerals include calcium, potassium, phosphorous and iron. They conserve their nutrients when raw. They should be eaten in moderation and without being fried. It is better to toast them lightly, cook them or crush them with sugar in order to produce a vegetable butter high in nutritional value. The oil retains its nutritional properties and has a pleasant taste.

**Therapeutic Indication:**  A general tonic for the organism. Reduces cholesterol due to its mono-saturated fat; useful against intestinal inflammation and colic of the kidneys and liver; it decreases the formation of tumors due to its linoleic acid, a fatty acid of the Omega 3 group. Exaggerated consumption may cause allergies or problems of the gallbladder and the pancreas, due to its high content of fat that can not be absorbed.

**Chestnuts**. An essential source of food for nutrition. They contain proteins, 2% fat, carbohydrates between 10% and 20%, and vegetable fibers that the body does not absorb, although they do contain a high proportion of minerals that are easy to absorb, such as potassium, phosphorous, calcium, magnesium and iron. They do not have many vitamins, the only ones being vitamin A and variable quantities of B1, B2 and B3.

**Therapeutic Indication:**   Reconstitutes the body; an excellent muscular tonic and restorer; it is astringent; useful for diarrhea and anemia in children; it is digestive and caloric; an excellent food for breast-feeding mothers.

**Flax seed**. Contains 27 anticancerigenous components, such as lignin, the content of which is more than 100 times that of whole grain. Contains essential polyunsaturated acids: 57% Omega 3, 16% Omega 6, 9% saturated and 18% monounsaturated fatty acids.  It is a nutritional food that has mucilaginous properties.

**Therapeutic Indication:** Helps to remove cholesterol; prevents high blood pressure, coagulation of the blood and heart attacks; regulates glucose; prevents cancer of the colon, breast cancer, prostate cancer, and lungs cancer; lubricates the digestive system and eases constipation; prevents colitis, arthritis and gastritis; strengthens the immune system; helps the nervous system; increases vitality, energy and is a natural aphrodisiac; unblocks the arteries; reduces appetite and is excellent for loosing weight. When eaten in the morning it maintains sugar levels in the blood.

**Walnuts**. An excellent food and to make it complete you can combine it with fruits such as apples and grapes. Its percentage of nutrients depends on the variety. They contain linoleic acid that is a fatty acid of the Omega 3 group, as well as 59% fat, proteins, carbohydrates, calories, vitamins A, C, B1 and B3, and calcium, iron, phosphorous and traces of magnesium and sulfur.

**Therapeutic Indication:** They are thermal and have preventive effect on cardiovascular diseases; invigorate the nervous system; activate the cerebral function;  act in cellular regeneration; invigorate the sexual function; useful against rheum and skin infections; Useful for old people as a liquefied vegetable milk with honey and water. External use: The oil may be applied on the skin to soften it, nourish it and make it more beautiful.

**Pine nuts**. Contain proteins, fats, carbohydrates, minerals and vitamins. Pine nut milk is made by blending pine nuts with honey and water.

**Therapeutic Indication:** They are thermal and act as a gentle laxative. They are digestive, reduce inflammation and act against allergies.

**Pistachio nuts**. Contain proteins, fats, carbohydrates, minerals and vitamins.

**Therapeutic Indication:** Thermal: remove parasites from the intestine; a smooth laxative; acts on the respiratory system and reduces inflammation.

# 5. PRODUCTS OF ANIMAL ORIGIN.

## Yoghurt.

A basic source of food in Turkey and Bulgaria, from where it is originated, produced by the fermentation of milk. It has lactic acid that propitiates intestinal flora, neutralizes and regulates secretion of acids in the stomach. It provides sufficient calcium, phosphorous and B complex and C vitamins, plus magnesium, zinc, protein and lecithin. It is refreshing and an easily digestible source of food, recommended for anyone who has intestinal problems, skin problems and problems of the nervous system. Its daily consumption as part of a vegetarian diet is recommended because the organism does not produce vitamin B12 and yoghurt has this vitamin.

Yoghurt is very tasty without sugar and you may add fruit if you wish. You can make it at home so that the lactobacillus acidophilus bacteria multiply better.

**How to make yoghurt**: You need one liter of milk, three heaped tablespoons of powdered milk and half a cup of plain yoghurt. Boil the milk and allow to cool until it is slightly warm (test it with your finger). Blend the milk with yoghurt and powdered milk at low speed for one minute. Add the remainder of the milk and stir well. Cover the receptacle and wrap it in a wool cloth to keep the temperature at $37^0$C for five hours or place it near the pilot light of the stove. It is better if you use a clay receptacle or if you cover it with a clay plate, so as to retain heat. When curdled, refrigerate.

## Curd cheese

**Preparation**: Use two liters of milk and four tablespoons of lime juice. Heat the milk and when it comes to boil, turn down the gas and add lime juice. Use a wooden spoon to gently stir the milk until it separates into lumps of curd cheese and whey. The whey should be clear, if not, add more lime juice. Turn out the gas. Place a thin piece of cloth in a strainer and pour the curd cheese over it to strain it. Hold the edges of the cloth to make a bag, rinse the curd under water, hang or place something heavy on it so that it strains completely. Leave for fifteen minutes to two hours.

## Cheese

The origin of cheese is unknown, although it had been known as "slices of milk" since the times of Homer. It started out as an artisan product but its basic preparation process has not changed. If you leave milk in the open air for certain time it becomes naturally contaminated, coagulates and ferments. Now, as in the past, various types of milk are used (cow's milk, sheep's milk or goat's milk). The modern industrial system mixes these various types of milk that manipulates more precisely the action of microbes. Some cheeses are obtained by using the pressing system only and they contain vitamin C, but are low in fat. Traditional cheese are the most tasty. Make sure that cheese does not have any color. Moderation is the norm when eating cheese.

Their consistency depends on moisture; the less moist, the harder they are. Fat content is calculated on the basis of the percentage of dry material in the cheese and varies between 22% and 47%, depending on the type of milk, either whole milk or low-fat milk. Milk's protein content ranges between 7% and 35% and has calcium and phosphorous in variable portions. Fresh cheese does not ripen. The ripening time of cheese may be natural or microbial when adding bacteria or mold. They ripen in damp or dry places, depending on the type of cheese.

**Cheese is divided into fresh, semi-hard and hard cheese.**

Fresh cheese: does not ripen and has a high moisture content. It should be kept refrigerated and be eaten promptly. These are the most recommended because they easily digested. The most popular are: panela, curd cheese, Oaxaca, ranchero, Burgos, cream cheese, etc.

Ripe cheese: manchego, Chihuahua, gruyer, cheddar, edam, Roquefort, goat cheese, camembert, brick and gorgonzola.

Hard cheese: compact and crumbly; for grating

The cheeses with the highest calorie content are cheddar, parmesan, cream, gruyer, camembert, etc.

## Milk

Mother's milk has been irreplaceable as man's first source of food. The best milk for human consumption is naturally homogenized goat's milk, because it is easy to assimilate.

Untreated cow's milk has enzymes that help digestion and produce less mucosities, although it does have microorganisms that damage the organism, therefore it should be boiled. Industrially-processed milk is heated and bacteria are removed using controlled and prescribed hygienic methods.

**<u>The risks of dairy products</u>**:  It is better not to consume dairy products in excess. The small intestine does not have the lactase and rennin enzymes needed to obtain milk's calcium. The function of the lactase and rennin enzymes is to split the two lactose molecules into glucose and galactose; if this is not done, then it ferments. European people have these enzymes. Adults and children who can not tolerate lactose substitute normal milk with skim milk, calcium and vitamins A, E, or B2, yoghurt or soy milk.

High consumption of dairy products is linked with: respiratory afflictions, asthma, hay fever, migraine, cardiac disease, cancer, arthritis, allergies, ear infection, intestinal inflammation, flatulence or diarrhea.

The only animal that drinks milk after weaning is Man.

## Eggs

The size or color of chicken eggs do not alter their nutritional value. The **eggshell** is pure calcium. The **egg white** contains albumin and half of the egg's protein. The **egg yolk** should be compact and in the middle of the egg white. It contains the remaining proteins, lecithin, vitamins A, B, D and E, iron, sulfur and is low in calories. Eggs are a nutritional source of food that are perfectly balanced and that contain the eight essential amino acids in ideal proportion. These are very important as they can not be produced by our organism, therefore, we must obtain them by eating certain types of food.

Children should eat eggs frequently. People suffering from ulcers or gout should eat eggs in moderation. People suffering from arteriosclerosis or who have a high level cholesterol should not eat eggs as the yolk has high content of cholesterol.

**In order to obtain natural calcium from the shell,** wash it well, remove the membrane, and dry and Blend until obtaining a powder. Take the tip of a teaspoon every day with meals.

Submerge eggs in salt water to make sure that they are fresh. If they sink horizontally they are fresh; if they sink vertically they are not so fresh, and if they float they are too old and should not be eaten.

## Bee's honey

Produced by bees from the pollen extracted from flowers. The world's vegetation gives us a wide variety of flowers, depending on the earth, weather, altitude and season. The honey of each country reflects the flowers from which it is produced. Honey has two types of sugars: glucose or dextrose and levulose or fructose.

Glucose is quickly digested and provides energy and levulose that is stored by the liver as a reserve in the form of glycogen.

Bee's honey contains organic acids and volatile substances that stimulate the appetite.

Minerals: phosphorous, calcium, iron, copper and manganese; all vitamins in small quantities; **enzymes**: invertase, a tonic against intestinal slowness and that has a catalytic action on the metabolism, and amylase, very effective for the peristaltic movement of the intestine and is needed for the metabolism of the honey's sugars, in addition to which it has all indispensable elements for preserving the organism's tissues.

**Nutritional value**: 100 grams of honey is equivalent to five eggs, 0.6 liters of milk, three bananas, four oranges, 120 grams of nuts and 78 grams of cheese.

**Therapeutic Indication**: Honey is an antibiotic, contains the "inhibin" of bacterial action and has active bacterial germs. It increases the amount of hemoglobin in the blood; it is effective for inflammations and infections of the respiratory tracts and of the mouth and the throat, etc.; it is an effective cure for stomach and gastric ulcers; it is a hepatic stimulant; it removes toxic waste from the urine; it acts an antiseptic for skin injuries. Linden honey calms the nervous system. It is slightly soporific and stimulates the digestion; it is diuretic and calms painful menstruation. Orange honey has a calming effect and is antispasmodic. Heather honey helps against gout, rheum and is very high in basic minerals. Wasp honey is excellent.

**Royal jelly:** Produced by bees for the queen bee. It is of high nutritional value, provides strength and longevity and contains vitamins, minerals and the essential amino acids that the organism needs. It is recommended for physical, intellectual and sexual exhaustion, premature aging, nervous depression, and menopause. It is also effective for treating sores, ulcers, herpes, gangrene, hepatitis, stomatitis and dermatitis (eczema).

**Propolis:** Bees take a sweet-smelling resin from the bark of certain trees that they use to seal their beehives and disinfect all germs.

**Therapeutic indications:** For the human body it is effective as a natural antibiotic in treating infections of the respiratory system. It has preventive action and strengthens the immune system, aids digestion, and the genital-urinary system and the dermatologic system. It regulates the endocrine glands; protects against telluric radiation (bees look for telluric crosses, use them and protect themselves with the bee glue that they produce).

**Bee pollen:** An invaluable source of nutrients for human health. It balances and invigorates. It is a complex mixture of the secretion of bees and flower pollen. Bees visit over 1000 flowers a day to collect nectar for making honey and pollen.

**Flower pollen:** The male seed of plants, present in the male sexual organs of flowers. It is a concentrated and complete source of food with a low moisture content that makes it stable and means that it may be preserved for a long time.

It is very rich in amino acids of vegetable origin and is of high biological value. Includes vitamins D, E, B, K, P (rutine) and pro-vitamin A, plus sodium, potassium, magnesium, calcium, aluminum, iron, copper and zinc. Enzymes include amylase, catylase, diaphorase, diastase, pectase, phosphotase and others. It also has fats, carbohydrates, fatty acids, oligoelements and high antibiotic power.

**Therapeutic Indication:** Helps the nervous and endocrine system; increases appetite and regulates intestinal functions; prevents the proliferation of harmful germs and infections of all types, as well as asthma and allergies, prostatis, rheumatism, diabetes and convalescence; stimulates the function of the liver and increases red blood cells; regulates intestinal flora; provides energy; invigorates and improves the function of various organs of the body; maintains the intellectual functions of the brain. It is a potent source of food for people with nutritional problems. It is a nutritional supplement that restores and revitalizes the organism.

The following recipe is for a very energetic source of food recommended for people who suffer from weakness.  Mix:

½ liter of honey

1 small jar of royal jelly

100 grams of bee glue

250 grams of pollen from shiny flowers

Stir in a glass jar and leave for twenty-one days. Take a teaspoon in the morning and half a teaspoon at night.

The ingredients in your kitchen

1. You

2. Love and patience

3. Familiarizing yourself with the cooking utensils you are going to use

4. An intimate encounter with fruit, grains, vegetables, etc.

5. A sense of gratitude and respect towards them.

6. Veneration for our Mother Earth.

7. Knowing what you want to do and how you are going to do it.

8. Start by doing what takes the longest.

9. Cook with happiness.

10. Be creative, invent your own dishes!

11. Get rid of useless things.

12. Do not waste anything.

13. Success is guaranteed! A healthy way of life for you and your family.


## Condiments

**Savory**. Used raw to accompany some salads. Stimulates digestion, regulates contractions of the intestine and prevents fermentation, benefiting the evacuation of gas. Drink as a tea to double its effect.

**Garlic**. A major ingredient for all types of foods. An excellent intestinal disinfectant and an excellent tonic of the organism. It is a natural antibiotic, purifies the blood, is a stimulant for the sexual function and propitiates the production of semen.

**Sweet basil**. May be used as a condiment. It is aromatic and sweet. Much used in Italian cooking for pastas, cheese soufflé, with tomatoes and steamed vegetables. It is diuretic, emmenagogue and carminative.

**Capers**. Capers are the buds of watercress and may be used to complement various types of dishes.

**Caraway**. A condiment that stimulates digestive function. Much used in Europe as is choucroute, curry, couscous, etc.

**Anise**. Used as an essence to aromatize cakes. It is stomachic and may be used to make tea, punch, sweets, oatmeal, etc.

**Cinnamon**. Used as spice. It is also an excellent tonic. It is sudorific. Aids digestion and acts against gases. To relieve colds, take as a tea with lime as this help sweating.

**Onion**. Used as condiment and medicine. Purifies the blood and stimulates production of blood. It helps to clean the liver, aids digestion and removes mucosa, and relieves earache, colds, dizziness, fever, etc. It is best eaten raw but in moderation by people suffering from ulcers, high pressure and colitis. Raw onion, garlic and ginger together increase their curative properties.

**Chives**. A taste similar to that of onion, although lighter and more delicate.

**Cilantro**. Has an intense aroma. Used as an aromatic and medicinal herb. Its seeds are used to season food and you may use it to make a tea that you can drink before meals as an appetizer, or after meals to aid digestion.

**Cloves**. Have a strong taste and should be used prudently for seasoning stews, sauces, etc. Acts as a tonic.

**Cumin**. Use as a condiment. Is an excellent stimulant and helps the stomach and digestive system. May be drunk as a tea and combined with other herbs, such as anis.

**Curcuma**. Pleasant and healthy; helps to prevent diabetes and cancer; excellent for the articulation, skin and mucus membranes, particularly of the female organs.

**Curry**. A mixture of spices, curcuma, coriander seed, ginger, thyme, cumin, paprika, and pepper. Served to season eggs, mayonnaise, stews, etc.

**Juniper**. An excellent condiment for some dishes. It is diuretic and antiseptic.

**Dill**. Aromatic. Used for cabbage, beetroots, cucumber, etc salads and for seasoning and bread.

**Mexican tea**. Use to give beans flavor; it is anthelmintic and emmenagogue. Tea drunk after eating aids digestion. Pregnant women may drink it in moderation.

**Tarragon**. Of Mongol origin. It has a sweet aroma and may be used to season, salads, sauces and stews. It is used for seasoning vegetable, etc., in salt-free diets It is digestive, contains an essential oil, stragol, that has an appetizing action.

**Fenugreek**. The seeds are used. It is an excellent laxative. Soak a teaspoon of seeds and three prunes in a glass of water overnight and drink in the morning.

**Gentian**. An excellent appetizer as it increases the secretion of saliva and gastric glands. Dissipates spasms and invigorates the nerves.

**Mint**. Has a delicious and sweet aroma. It is digestive, a general stimulant, antispasmodic sedative, improves the appetite, and relieves intellectual fatigue and sexual insufficiency. Its effect is doubled when taken as a tea.

**Fennel**. It is an appetizer, stomachic, carminative and emmenagogue. Only the leaves and stalks are used; the seeds may be used to aromatize some cakes.

**Ginger**. "Man without ginger loses his strength and his woman" says an ancient Chinese proverb. Ginger root is used as herb and as a form of medication. It is a stimulant for the digestion, a cerebral tonic, nourishes the nervous system and the bronchi, and eases fatigue and fever.

**Bay leaves**. Many cultures use it for different purposes, such as a celebratory crown, for protection, fortune telling, etc. It gives a sweet aroma to culinary preparations. When you have seasoned your stews, soups, etc, remove the leaves. Digestive. When taken as a teas it eases chronic bronchitis. The oil of its seeds is an excellent balsam against rheumatism.

**Lime**. It is alkalinizing, disinfectant, stimulates the liver, and dissolves uric acid and mucosity. It is a source of vitamin C, calcium, potassium, magnesium, etc. Lime juice with honey in hot water is excellent for breaking a fast. Cleans the throat and stomach of mucus in the event of colds.

**Panch Masala**. With whole grains in equal parts: cumin seed, black cumin or kalinji, black mustard, anise, or fenugreek. Place the herbs in a hermetically sealed container, place in a cool, dark and dry place; stir the jar before using the ingredients.

**Garam Masala**. Toast separately: four teaspoons of coriander grain and two teaspoons of each one: cumin in grain, cloves, cardamom seeds and two sticks of cinnamon 5 cm. long. Grind until producing a fine powder and keep in a cool place.

**Marjoram**. Has a strong aroma and a sweet taste. Commonly used for Italian dishes, soups and stews. It is stomachic, diuretic, a stimulant, calms the nervous system and infections of the liver. Taken as a tea it calms nervous tics, and relieves asthma, acute or chronic catarrh, bronchitis and coughs.

**Mustard**. France made this famous in the Dijon region. Mixed with vinegar and other aromatizings it may be used to accompany various types of dishes and sauces. Stimulates the functioning of the pancreas and the suprarenal glands, and facilitates digestion. Do not eat too much. The main problem with mustard is its chemical origin and it may cause damage. To treat colds and pain, apply ¼ of mustard flour and ¾ of flaxseed flour as a poultice.

**Nutmeg**. A condiment used for many sweets and dishes. It is a stimulant for the digestive system and the general condition of the organism.

**Oregano**. It is similar to marjoram, but with a more intense flavor. It is used to alleviate intestinal infection, amebiasis and dysentery.

**Paprika**. A multi-use condiment. Excellent for the memory.

**Parsley**. The legend says that whoever planted parsley must have been a good and fair man. Rich in minerals such as iron and calcium, and has various oligoelements and vitamin C. It is excellent for reconstituting the blood, helps in the treatment of diabetes, cleans the kidneys, reduces birth pain and menstruation and reduces hemorrhages. It is anti-abortive and regulates the balance of calcium in the organism. It is diuretic, cholagogue, sedative, emmenagogue and aphrodisiacal. Its juice may be used to treat poisoning. Chew parsley after eating garlic. It is very fragile and become oxidized rapidly when coming into contact with light. Preserve it by wrapping it in aluminum foil. Parsley root eaten in large quantities may cause poisoning.

**Pepper**. The world's most popular herb. It may be the best or the worst, depending on how it is used. If eaten in large quantities it wears down the taste buds and causes sweating and irritation in the stomach mucus. Normal consumption aids digestion. It is aphrodisiacal.

**White pepper** is the ripened fermented fruit not dried in the sun. **Black pepper** is the ripe and fermented fruit and dried in the sun. **Green pepper** is when the grain is green. **Red pepper** is white or black pepper but without being fermented. It may be used in stews, soups, etc. and improves the flavor of the main ingredient. **Pink pepper** is the seeds of the pirul. Dry and crushed papaya seeds may be used as a replacement for pepper.

**Horseradish**. Similar to the turnip. An ingredient used for mustard. Used in sauces with cream, stews, etc.

**Rosemary**. It is said that it is cultivated to attract gnomes. It has a strong aroma and a bitter-sweet and hot taste. It brings out the aroma of any sauce or dish. It aids digestion and eliminates gas. It is antirheumatic and invigorating, regulates menstruation and calms the nerves. It aids in infections and healing wounds.

**Sage**. Sage (also called the tea of Provenza) has many virtues and for the Romans it was sacred. It has a strong taste and is slightly bitter. It should be used in small quantities and added at the last moment of cooking. Activates blood circulation, and prevents transpiration; protects life and helps to give life; purifies, invigorates the stomach and activates the kidneys and the liver. The properties and aroma of sage tea are much greater than many others. Sage, broom, boldo and cedron tea drunk before breakfast is excellent for the liver.

**Stevia (Rebaudina)**. An herb with unusual leaves that are thirty times sweeter than any common sugar, with the advantage that it does not have any calories, as it is a non-metabolic sweetener, in other words, it does not remain in the organism. It not only has a sweet taste, but also therapeutic properties, the most important beings its hypoglycemia effect.

**Thyme**. It has been used for centuries. It has a strong and penetrating taste and aroma and is used for all types of stews, soups, cheese sauces, etc. It has an essential oil called thymol. It is more effective as a tea, relieving physical digestion, fermentation, gas and intestinal inflammation, lack of appetite, cardiac weakness, anemia, physical and intellectual fatigue, neurasthenia, cough, bronchial infections (asthma, bronchitis), colds, insomnia, hepatic disorders and urinary infections.

**Vanilla**. It has a smooth and delicious taste and flavor. May be used for sweets, puddings, biscuits, etc.

**Vinegar**. Not recommended because it causes acidity, dissolves hemoglobin of the blood and weakens the body's defenses.

**Apple vinegar.** Alkaline and helps to conserve the humidity of the intestine. How to prepare: One liter of water, one stick of concentrated sugar (piloncillo) and three diced apples with the peel and core removed. Place in a glass jar, cover and leave for seven days. Strain and place in the refrigerator.

# OILS.

Sunflower, corn, olive, sesame seed, flaxseed oils. Preferably consume virgin oils (cold pressed).

For frying:  olive oil, peanut oil and butter.

For salads: olive oil, flaxseed oil, avocado oil and walnut oil.

# PRACTICAL TIPS

## At meal times

- Eat calmly and without being upset, thus avoiding digestive problems.

- Eat happily and in peaceful surroundings.

- Eat only when you are hungry and chew and salivate food well.

- Do not eat after an emotional shock, because the transformation of food is unbalanced.

- Eat raw food with every meal.

- Salad is basic. It should be served as an entrée to improve the appetite, aid digestion and prevent thirst during the meal.

- Drink a little water during meals because it dilutes gastric juice.

- Do not eat between meals, just drink fruit juices.

- Do not eat fresh mushrooms more than one or twice a week.

- Present your meals attractively. Take distribution into account as well as combination of colors, cleanliness and order.

- When you need to sweet your meals, use bee's honey, maguey honey, maple syrup, molasses and brown sugar.

- Do not eat any high-fat cakes or sweets.

## When cooking

People who like cooking say that the kitchen is the heart of the house, where you should cook in pleasant and practical surroundings with utensils and ingredients at hand.

- Utensils should be made of stainless steel or spelter that is not chipped.

- Use large, medium-sized and small knives with a serrated and well-sharpened edge.

- Cook using seasonal products. They are the most abundant and economical.

- Vary your meals daily to obtain a balanced diet.

- Do not overcook vegetables; they should remain almost raw cooked. Cook on a low flame and use a little water so that they do not lose their nutritional properties.

- Cooking water should not be thrown away; you can use it for soups, etc.

- Combine the various dishes of a meal so that they compensate.

- Replace cane vinegars with lime or use apple vinegar.

- To improve vinegar, add orange peel, piquín chile, garlic, papaya seeds and leave for a week.

- Do not eat canned food.

- Avoid fried food as much as possible.

- Raw potatoes absorb salt.

- To avoid crying when cutting onion, slice it into a receptacle with water in it. Scrub the cutting board with half a lime so that it does not retain the smell of onion.

- To remove the strong flavor of cabbage, onion, etc, spray with very hot water, lime juice and salt. If you added too much salt, to a stew add thick slices of onion and leave for thirty minutes.

- The unpleasant odor given off by cauliflower and cabbage when boiled may be avoided by adding sugar to the water or a slice of bread.

- In order to make it easier to peel cloves of garlic, crush with a knife or soak them in hot water for a few seconds, after which the peel may easily be removed.

- Keep your garlic for as long as you wish. Place peeled cloves of garlic in a glass jar and add olive oil. Cover and refrigerate. The oil may be used as a garnish for salads and bread.

- Add olives to your normal oil and you will have olive oil handy for emergencies.

- You may crush any leftovers of cheese with parsley, garlic, estragon, thyme and salt and use them for stuffing poblano peppers, red tomatoes or red, green or yellow pepper.

- If you want to save your peppers, grill them and then clean them and spread with oil.

- In order to obtain more juice from lemons, place them in boiling water with the peel for five minutes.

- Remove stalks or green parts on potatoes before preparing them.

- When cooking without salt, season your dishes with tomato, green pepper, lime juice, diced onion and bay leaves, or with sliced onion, salvia, thyme, marjoram, curry and oregano.

- The taste of your vegetable dishes will be improved by adding spicy herbs. Traditional herbs include bay leaves, marjoram and thyme, but you may use your own combinations of oregano, parsley, mint, celery. Do not use too much and use less hot spices such as pepper, mustard, etc. Use bay leaves and saffron in small quantities.

- Keep your cooking herbs in a cool, dry place so that they do not loose their flavor.

- If fruit is still not ripe, wrap it in paper and let it ripen at room temperature.

- Ripe cantaloupes may have yellow, not green, peel. Shake honeydew melons and if the pits move freely it is ripe.

- Peel and wash fruit and vegetables under hot water before eating.

- Rinse raisins and dry fruit in hot water before eating.

- Cover raisins with flour so that they do not go to the bottom of cakes.

- Replace milk cream with natural yoghurt that is high in calcium with bacteria that ensures excellent intestinal flora.

- Agar is obtained from sea algae and is a mucilaginous substance used for substituting grenetine.

- Defrost food slowly. Ice breaks the balance of the food, producing changes in its structure and properties, which influence in its quality.

- Cayenne chili (piquín) and habanero chili have therapeutic properties. Cayenne chili stimulates blood circulation and cures gastric ulcers.

- Dijon mustard is a replacement for egg yolk.

- Grate beetroot to adorn your plate.

- Cover peeled apples with oil and lime to avoid oxidation.

- Croutons: leftovers of bread. Fry with garlic, parsley and salt.

## There are several methods for disinfecting fruits and vegetables:

- To remove insect or worm eggs add one tablespoon of salt per liter of water.

- You may remove bacteria and fungus by adding water with a few drops of permanganate tincture (an excellent antiseptic) and leave them to soak for ten minutes. Then wash well and place in clean water with lime juice and a little salt. Note: if permanganate comes in the form crystals, just place a few on the tip of a knife in one liter of water and leave overnight. Use one spoonful of this mixture for every liter of water.

- Use five drops of iodine tincture for every two liters of water.

- To release germs from root vegetables and fruits, place them in boiling water and then in cold water and repeat the process.

- With a few drops of lemon juice.

## Method of preparing whole meal rice:

1 cup of brown rice

2 cloves of garlic

¼ diced or sliced onion

2 stalks of diced celery .

3 cups of vegetable broth or water.

Add salt.

Wash the rice well and boil for three minutes. Rinse with cold water and drain. Fry lightly in a little oil with the onion and garlic. Add water, celery and salt. When coming to the boil, cover and cook on a low gas for forty-five minutes. Do not take the lid off the saucepan while cooking.

# **60** Menus

# Menu # 1

**Hindu salad**
**Potato and sleek soup**
**Stuffed peppers**

### Hindu salad
2  chopped or grated cucumbers
2  grated carrots
1  tbs. of turnip seeds
4  tbs. of chopped parsley
1  cup of yogurt
   Salt and pepper to taste
Blend yogurt with cucumber peel and condiment with salt and pepper. Mix all ingredients. Very refreshing.

### Potato and sleek soup
½ kg of sliced potatoes
½ cup of chopped leek
1 red tomato (optional)
¼ onion
1 clove of garlic
1 liter of vegetable broth or water
2 tbs. of oil
Grill red tomato and blend with onion and garlic; season in oil. Add broth, potatoes and leek. Simmer until potatoes are cooked.

### Stuffed peppers
6  grill red bell peppers
   Salt, pepper and nutmeg to taste
4  medium-size potatoes, cooked and chopped
200 grams of chopped walnut
100 grams of pine nuts
100 grams of white raisins
½  cup of chopped parsley
3  tbs. of olive oil
50 grams of walnut
1  cup of milk
2  eggs
Salt to taste
Wash peppers and sprinkle them with salt, pepper and nutmeg. Lightly condiment potatoes, walnut, pine nuts, raisins and parsley in oil. Stuff peppers with this mixture. Beat egg white to a nougat-like consistency and add yolks. Cover peppers with flour, dip in the egg and fry. Blend remaining walnut with milk and salt. Bathe peppers in this sauce.
Note: If you do not want to use egg, dip the peppers in wheat germ. Serve with a teaspoon of mayonnaise. Delicious.

# Menu # 2

**Roquefort salad**
**Macaroni with Mexican squash**
**Ratatouille**

## Roquefort salad

½ Romaine lettuce, washed and dried
½ escarole lettuce, washed and dried
½ cucumber
1 cup of fresh chopped spinach
2 tbs. of chopped parsley
1 red tomato
¼ sliced onion
¼ cup of lightly roasted pine nuts
   Sliced Roquefort cheese
   Salt to taste

Disinfect vegetables. Break lettuces into pieces by hand. Mix the vegetables and put in a serving dish; sprinkle with vinaigrette dressing to taste. Garnish with pine nuts and cheese.

## Macaroni with Mexican squash

300 grams of macaroni
2 sliced Mexican squash (zucchini)
2 sliced yellow peppers
2 dry-fried and ground red tomatoes
5 tbs. of olive oil
1 tbs. of whole wheat flour
 Parsley to taste

Cook macaroni in water with salt and a little oil and leave *al dente*; drain and sprinkle with oil. Sauté the pepper for two minutes, add the Mexican squash and squash flower. Cook for another two minutes, add tomato and condiment with salt and pepper. Sprinkle the flour and cook for 5 minutes. Put the pasta in a serving dish and bathe with Mexican squash sauce.

## Ratatouille

½ kg of eggplant diced in cubes
½ kg of Mexican squash cut into slices
½ kg of peeled and chopped red tomato
1 chopped bell pepper,
2 cloves of garlic, crushed and chopped
1 large chopped onion
1 tsp. of chopped basil
1 tsp. of oregano
   Salt to taste

Place vegetables in a saucepan in layers and condiment with basil, oregano and salt. Sprinkle with a little water and cover. Cook on a low heat for 30 minutes.

3 Cups of finely chopped squash flower
    Salt and pepper to taste

# Menu # 3

**Garlic broccoli**
**Tapioca soup**
**Aztec cake**

## Garlic broccoli

1 kg of broccoli
½ cup of cooked French beans (optional)
3 tbs. of olive oil
3 chopped cloves of garlic
¼ cup of chopped walnut
1 chopped Julienne bell pepper
1 lime (juice)
  Salt to taste

Cook broccoli in a little boiling water with salt and half the lime juice for 8 minutes on a low heat. Remove from heat and drain. Lightly fry garlic, pepper, French beans, broccoli and lime juice in olive oil for 4 minutes. Remove from heat and sprinkle with walnut.

## Tapioca soup

1 cup of tapioca or one handful per person
2 tbs. of corn oil
½ cup of grated carrots
¼ cup of grated turnip
½ cup of milk
1 tbs. of chopped mint (optional)
1 tbs. of chopped coriander (optional)
  Salt to taste

Soak the tapioca overnight. Use the same water to cook the tapioca and then add milk. When it starts boiling, add vegetables and condiment with salt. When tapioca becomes transparent, add oil, mint and coriander and stir. Cover the saucepan, turn out the heat and stand.

## Aztec cake

18 corn tortillas
6 washed and grill poblano peppers
6 tender corns, with the grain removed and cooked
4 cups of chopped squash flowers
4 chopped Mexican squash
5 chopped cloves of garlic
2 chopped onions
4 chopped large red tomatoes,
200 grams of grated Chihuahua cheese
200 grams of fresh or goat cheese
1 cup of yogurt (to taste)
¼ cup of mayonnaise.
  Oil as needed
  Salt to taste

Cut chilies into strips. Sauté garlic, onion, corn, peppers, red tomato, Mexican squash, and squash flower. Cook for 10 minutes at low heat. Remove and let stand. Lightly fry the tortillas in oil. Grate both cheeses together. Place a layer of tortillas in a dish, then a layer of vegetables, a layer of cheese and a layer of yogurt (mix the yogurt with the mayonnaise) until you end up with cheese and yogurt. Cover the dish with tinfoil. Place in a regular oven for 20-25 minutes. Serve hot.

# Menu # 4

**Avocado salad**
**Pearl barley soup**
**Curried French beans with soy milk**

## Avocado salad

3  avocados
1  lime (juice)
2  chopped spring onions
1  handful bundle of chopped coriander
3  washed and grill poblano peppers
100 grams of grated Chihuahua or ripe cheese
1  tbs. of olive oil
   Salt to taste

Peel avocados, cut into squares and sprinkle with lime juice. Mix with coriander, onion and strips of chili. Garnish with cheese. Serve with rye bread.

## Pearl barley soup

6  tbs. of pearl barley, soaked
1  sliced leek
2  chopped celery stems
1  large red tomato, ground raw
2  cloves of garlic
2  tbs. chopped parsley
2  tbs. chopped coriander
2  tbs. olive oil
6 cups of vegetable broth or water
   Salt to taste

Cook barley in broth; when tender, add remaining ingredients and let boil until the leek is cooked.

## Curried French beans

½  kg of French beans soaked for 12 hours
½  kg of string beans, cut into pieces
1  chopped onion
2  chopped cloves of garlic
1  red pepper, in thin slices
1 ½  tsp. of turmeric
1 ½  tsp. of grated cumin
1  tsp of ginger powder
1  tsp of ground coriander seeds
4  tbs. of oil
2  cloves of spice
1  tsp. of cardamom
¼  cup of soy milk
Salt to taste

Cook French beans on a low heat in the water they were soaked in and then drain. Sauté the garlic, onion, pepper, cardamom, cloves and string beans in the oil. Add French beans and stir constantly. Add the rest of the ingredients, salt and a little of the broth in which the French beans were cooked. Season for 10 minutes, and stir occasionally to prevent soy milk from sticking to the sides of the saucepan. Remove cloves and cardamom grains before serving.
Note: Can be accompanied with whole rice instead of barley soup.

# Menu # 5

**Green broad bean salad**
**Oats soup**
**Salsify stew**

**Green broad bean salad**
¾   kg of cooked green broad beans
2    avocados, cut in stripes
1    chopped red bell pepper
1    tbs. of olive oil
     Salt and oregano to taste
Mix all ingredients

**Oats soup**
½    cup of oats
½    cup of chopped sleek
1    cup of chopped garlic
1    sprig of mint
8    cups of vegetable broth or water
4    tbs. of oil
¼    tbs. of chopped turnip,
¼    cup of chopped celery with leaves
1    tbs. of chopped onion
1    chopped xoconoxtle without the seeds
     Salt to taste

Sauté the garlic, onion and vegetables in oil; add water or broth. When half cooked, add the oats and simmer for 5 minutes. Add salt and mint. Stand before serving.

**Salsify stew**
1    kg. of salsify, cooked and peeled
1    sliced pepper
2    chopped red tomatoes,
1    onion, Julienne style or to taste
2    tbs. of chopped garlic
4    tbs. of oil
     Aromatic herbs
     Salt to taste
Sauté garlic and onion in oil. Add salsify, tomato and pepper. Condiment with salt and aromatic herbs. Cook at a low heat. Remove, cover and stand.

# Menu # 6

**Walnut salad**
**Rice with chard**
**Vegetable ragout**

**Walnut salad**
½   Romaine lettuce in pieces
½   French lettuce in  pieces
2    bundles of watercress, in pieces
3    sliced celery stems
225 grams of diced walnuts

**Dressing**
2    tbs. of apple vinegar
6    tbs. of olive oil
     Salt and pepper to taste
Disinfect vegetables. Mix and season with dressing. Garnish with walnuts.

**Rice with chard**
1    cup of brown rice
4    cups of chopped chard
3    cups of vegetable broth or water
4    tbs. of chopped coriander
4    tbs. of chopped parsley
4    tbs. of oil
5    cloves of garlic
¼    chopped onion
     Sea salt to taste

Wash rice and cook in boiling water for 3 minutes; wash with cold water and drain. Fry rice in oil with garlic and onion. Add water, chard, coriander and salt. Cook at a low heat. When it begins to dry, add parsley. Total cooking time: 45 minutes or until cooked.

**Vegetable ragout**
¼    kg of chopped mushrooms
1    eggplant
1    chopped green Mexican squash
1    chopped yellow squash
1    chopped red or yellow pepper
2    chopped red tomatoes
1    chopped onion
5    chopped cloves of garlic
1    pinch of cinnamon powder
1    tbs. of chopped basil
¼    tsp. of ground cumin
3    tbs. of olive oil
     Sea salt and pepper to taste
Sauté in olive oil all ingredients. Cover and let season at a low heat for 10 minutes. Remove and let stand.

# Menu # 7

**Vinaigrette artichokes**
**Soy bean soup**
**Cabbage rolls with rice**

**Vinaigrette artichoke**
6    pieces of fresh artichokes, washed
6    lime slices
1½   of finely chopped chayote or red onion
1½   tbs. of Dijon mustard
¼    tbs. of thyme
2    tbs. of chopped fresh parsley
2    tbs. of chopped olives
3    tbs. of apple vinegar
6    tbs. of olive oil
Lime juice
Marine salt to taste
Cut artichoke stems and remove the hard leaves around the lower part. Cover base with a slice of lime and tie it with a piece of string. Place artichokes in hot water with salt and lime juice, and cook for 35 minutes. Once cooked, rinse in cold water and drain. Place mustard, thyme and vinegar in a bowl and blending with a mixer; add oil very slowly and continue mixing. Add parsley. Separate artichoke leaves and arranges them in a serving dish in an attractive manner. Remove out the heart from the base, remove the fibrous part and throw it away (do not try to eat it). Place the heart among the leaves and sprinkle with vinaigrette.

**Soy bean soup**
2    cups of cooked soy beans
2    grill and ground red tomatoes
1    crushed and chopped clove of garlic
¼    cup of chopped onion
¼    cup of chopped leek
4    tbs. of oil
1    pinch of cumin powder
     Soy sauce to taste
Blend beans in 6 cups of the water used to cook them and sieve. Sauté the garlic, onion, leek and tomato. Let season. Add beans and cook for 20 minutes at a low heat. Add soy sauce. Serve with croutons.

**Cabbage rolls with rice**
1    piece of medium-size cabbage
2    cups of cooked rice, preferably from the day before
1    chopped onion
     Salt to taste
1    cup of ground squash seeds
3    red tomatoes
1    Guajillo chili
1    Piquín chili (cayenne)
1    sprig of epazote
Cook cabbage with the leaves removed in water with salt, sugar, cumin, Bay leaves and cold bread. Remove bread and drain. Fry garlic and onion, add rice and cook for 3 minutes.
Sauce: Cook tomatoes with chilies, epazote and salt. Remove the epazote. Blend and sieve. Add squash seeds diluted in the water in which the tomatoes were cooked. Fry in oil. Let season. Stuff cabbages leaves with rice and place the rolls on a serving dish; bathe with the seed sauce. Serve with black bread

# Menu # 8

**Cucumber salad**
**Brgl wheat soup**
**Eggplant**

### Cucumber salad
2   finely chopped cucumbers,
¾   cup of jocoque (curdled milk)
4   cloves of garlic (juice)
1   tbs. of dry mint
    Sea salt and pepper to taste
Mix all ingredients. Season jocoque with garlic juice, salt and pepper. Sprinkle mint to garnish.

### Brgl wheat soup
2   cups of thick wheat soaked for ½ hour
5   cloves of garlic
300g of sliced panela cheese or vegetarian
  Cheese.
6   tbs. of olive oil
5   cups of water or vegetable broth
    Salt to taste
Fry the garlic in oil in a saucepan. Rinse and drain the wheat already soaked in hot water and add the broth to the garlic oil. Add salt when it comes to the boil, cover the saucepan and leave to simmer. When, almost cooked, place the cheese on top. Serve with jocoque or natural yogurt. Delicious!

### Eggplant
3   eggplants
¼   cup of apple vinegar
¾   cup of olive oil
2   chopped cloves of garlic
Salt to taste
Cut the eggplants into thick strips and marinate for 1-2 hours with the four other ingredients. Grill until brown; dice when cool.
Add:
1   chopped red onion,
2   tbs. of chopped olives
2   tbs. of chopped capers
    Sea salt and pepper to taste
To serve:
3   tbs. of fresh chopped basil

# Menu # 9

**Purslane salad**
**Broad bean soup**
**Green enchiladas**

### Purslane salad
2    cups of chopped tender purslane
1    cup of diced fresh pineapple
1    cup of diced jícama
½    chopped onion
½    tsp. of mustard (optional)
1    lime (juice)
1    pinch of cumin powder
     Olive oil to taste
     Salt to taste
Clean, wash and disinfect purslane and drain. Mix all ingredients and season. You may use your favorite dressing.

### Broad bean soup
½    kilo of dry broad beans
1    onion cut into quarters
1    chopped onion
2    red tomatoes
¼    tsp. of ground cumin
1    cup of chopped coriander
2    tbs. of oil
     Sea salt to taste
Soak broad beans for 24 hours. Cook in a pot with water and diced onion. Add the other ingredients half way through cooking, except the coriander, added when you turn out the heat. Let stand. Serve hot.

### Green enchiladas
12    tortillas
½     kilo of green tomatoes
½     cup of disinfected coriander
½     small onion
¼     cup of chopped onion
3     cloves of garlic
3     green chilies to taste
200 grams of cottage or panela cheese
100 grams of yogurt or cream
6of oil
 Sea salt to taste
Grind the green tomatoes, chilies, garlic, onion, and coriander raw. You may leave this sauce raw, or you can season it with a tablespoon of oil. Lightly sauté the tortillas and add them to the sauce.
Stuff with cottage cheese or garnish with onion slices.

# Menu # 10

**Beetroot salad**
**Onion soup**
**Soy in walnut sauce**

**Beetroot salad**

2    cups of raw cooked, diced or grated beetroot
½    cup of yogurt or to taste
1    tsp. of chopped onion
1    tsp. of chopped parsley

Place the beetroot on a serving dish, and add yogurt or, if you wish, mix both ingredients and garnish with onion and parsley.

**Onion soup**

1    sliced red onion
5    tbs. of olive oil
1    tbs. of brown sugar, or to taste
1    cinnamon stick
5    cups of vegetable broth
1    loaf of stale whole meal bread, diced
    Parmesan cheese to taste

Fry onion with sugar and cinnamon until brown. Add broth, cover, and simmer for 20 minutes. Add bread and let boil until it breaks up. Serve with Parmesan cheese. This homemade soup originates from Toscana Florence, in Italy.

**Soy in walnut sauce**

1    kilo of finely diced protoleg (textured soy) or wheat gluten
250 grams of walnut
¼    fried baguette
1onion
2large and ripe red tomatoes
2Seedless and toasted guajillo peppers
1Ancho chili pepper
2    tbs. of lightly toasted sesame seeds
1cinnamon stick
1aromatic clove
¼    of macho banana
3tbs. of oil
 Marine salt to taste

Boil all the herbs you have in water, and when boiling, add soy or gluten and let boil for another 10 minutes; then sieve and drain. Fry soy until brown. Blend remaining ingredients, sieve and lightly season in oil; add soy and salt. Let season together. A very tasty dish.

# Menu # 11

**Hawaiian salad**
**Dry pea soup**
**Oat croquettes**

## Hawaiian salad

100g  of mungo bean sprouts
  (called soy bean)
100g  of alfalfa sprouts
100g  of Wakame seaweed
2cups of diced fresh pineapple,
1banana

**Dressing**: mix the same amounts of apple vinegar and soy sauce; add honey to taste and the juice of one lime.

Place the sprouts in a serving dish to form a "bed". Wash the wakame seaweed in cold water and soak for 15 minutes. Drain, dice finely and spread on sprouts. Place banana slices and then the pineapple. Add dressing.

## Dry pea soup

1    cup of dry peas soaked for 12 hours
2    chopped carrots
½    sliced leek
½    chopped onion
5    cups of vegetable broth
¼    tbs. of thyme
½    tsp. of sweet basil
1    pinch of cumin
1    bay leaf
½    cup of light cream (optional)
     or natural yogurt.
     Sea salt to taste
     Croutons

Sauté the onion well, then add the carrots and spices. Cook in a covered saucepan on a low heat for one minute. Add peas and broth. Cook for 1½ hours partially covered at a low heat. Blend soup with yogurt. Serve hot with croutons.

## Oat Croquettes

1 ½ cups of oat flakes
½    cup of amaranth
½    chopped onion
4    tbs. of chopped coriander, or to taste
4    tbs. of chopped parsley, or to taste
2    eggs or garbanzo flour
Oil as necessary
Salt to taste

Mix oats, amaranth, onion, coriander, parsley and salt. Beat egg whites until a nougat-like consistency and add yolks (or garbanzo flour instead of eggs); then add vegetables and stir. Spoon separate portions into hot oil and fry croquettes on both sides until slightly brown. Drain on a cloth or napkins. Serve with garnish to taste.

# Menu # 12

**Asparagus**
**Saint Germain soup**
**Peppers stuffed with lentils**

### Asparagus

12    asparagus
¼    cup of clarified butter or
3 tbs. of sesame seed oil (optional)
3 tbs. of disinfected chopped parsley
2    eggs, cooked and chopped (optional)
6    chopped olives (optional)
Lime juice to taste
Salt to taste
Wash asparagus, cut off the hard part and cook for 6-7 minutes in a little water with salt and lime juice. Drain and place in a serving dish, add melted butter or sesame seed oil; then sprinkle with lime juice, parsley, and salt.

### Saint Germain soup

1 ½ cup of pearl barley in flakes
1    cup of sliced leek
1    cup of sliced celery
½    cup of grated carrot
5    cups of vegetable broth
4    tbs. of olive oil
Salt and pepper to taste
4    Slices of bread cut into squares
Oil for frying as necessary

Cook barley and vegetables in broth until they are "*al dente*" and blend one half. Cook all together at low heat, condiment with salt, and at initial boil turn fire off. Let it rest. Sauté bread. Serve hot, with croutons on top. Add flour to thicken the soup.

### Peppers stuffed with lentils

6    bell peppers
2    cups of cooked lentils
1    large chopped onion
2    cups of grated Cheddar cheese
2    cups of seasoned red tomato
1    cup of chopped walnut
4    tbs. of olive oil
     Swiss cheese to taste
     Salt to taste
Wash peppers, cut of the top part and remove the seeds and veins. Chop the veins and tops and remove stems. Steam for 3 minutes on a low heat. Sauté onion and chopped veins. Add drained lentils, cook for 3 minutes and add cheese until melted. Add sauce and walnuts and condiment to taste. Stuff peppers with this mixture. Place them in a greased tray and place small pieces of cheese piece on each pepper. Bake at 350º for 15-20 minutes.

# Menu # 13

**Watercress salad**
**Beetroot cream**
**Stuffed Poblano peppers with puff paste**

**Watercress salad**

2　cups of washed and chopped watercress
1　French lettuce
2　thinly sliced red tomatoes
1　thinly sliced onion
½　cup of chopped coriander
¼　cup of chopped almonds

**Dressing:**
1　avocado
2　cloves of garlic
2　tbs. of olive oil
　Juice of one lime
　Sea salt to taste

Disinfect vegetables and drain. Place the watercress, lettuce, onion and red tomato in a salad bowl. Blend a slice of onion, the garlic, avocado, salt, oil and lime juice. Bathe vegetables with the dressing and garnish with almonds.

**Beetroot soup**

¾　cup of wheat flour (semolina).
4　beetroots
½　sliced leek
6　cups of vegetable broth or water
5　tbs. of olive oil
　Sea salt to taste

Wash and scrub beetroots and cook with the peel in half of the broth. Sauté leek and semolina in oil and then add the rest of the broth and boil for 15 minutes.

Blend beetroots with the cooking broth and pour in the cooked semolina. Cook a few more minutes. Serve hot. You may add a tablespoon of yogurt and chopped parsley in the center of the dish.

**Stuffed Poblano peppers with puff paste**

6　poblano peppers grilled and washed
3　cups of cooked black beans
2　cups of huitlacoche
1　chopped onion,
2　crushed and chopped cloves of garlic
300 grams of cream cheese
1　cup of cream or natural yogurt
1　beaten egg
½　kilo of puff paste
6　tbs. of oil
Sesame seeds to taste
Salt to taste

Crush the beans and fry them in oil with half a chopped onion and salt. Lightly crush the huitlacoche and sauté with the rest of the onion, garlic and salt. Stuff peppers with beans and huitlacoche. Spread puff paste and roll until thin and then cut into squares. Place a stuffed pepper in each square and cover with the paste, pressing down firmly. Place in a flat oven dish, cover with the egg and sprinkle with sesame seeds. Bake at 350º until pastry is slightly brown. Blend yogurt with cream cheese and season. Bathe with cheese sauce to serve.

# Menu # 14

**Chayote salad**
**Vegetable minestrone**
**Tofu croquettes with salsify**

## Chayote salad

3      chayotes, peeled, cooked and diced
200 grams of fresh cheese
1      thinly sliced onion
3      tbs. of olive oil
½      tbs. of lime juice
1      tsp. of oregano powder
Soak onion in hot water with lime while chayotes are cooking. When cool, mix all ingredients and garnish with fresh cheese.

## Vegetable minestrone

3      diced eggplants
4      Mexican squash cut into thick strips
5      chopped red tomatoes
1      chopped onion
3      cloves of garlic
½      cup of vegetable broth
1      sprig of fresh rosemary
½      sprig of chopped basil
3      tbs. of grated Parmesan cheese
4      tbs. of olive oil
       Salt and pepper to taste
¼      kilo of whole pasta (to taste)
Soak eggplants in cold water for 10 minutes and drain. Sauté garlic and onion, add eggplant, Mexican squash, red tomato, broth, rosemary, pepper and salt and boil on a low heat for 10 minutes. Cook pasta separately in salted water and then throw away the cooking water. Mix vegetables, pasta, basil and cheese.

## Tofu croquettes with salsify

1      cup of salsify, cooked and diced into
       3 cm squares
1      tbs. of olive oil or butter
1      cup of diced leek (3 cm-pieces)
1      chopped onion,
1      chopped sprig of parsley, or to taste
300 grams of tofu (soy cheese)
1 egg or chickpea flour
2      tbs. of soy sauce
3      tbs. of chopped almonds or pistachios
2      tbs. of ground bread
2      tbs. of grated Parmesan cheese
1      tbs. of lime juice or apple vinegar
Salt and pepper to taste.
½      cup of vegetable broth
½      cup of yogurt
2      tbs. of chopped chives
Crush tofu with a fork and then mix with the onion, parsley, almonds, soy sauce, egg, bread, cheese, salt and pepper. Knead into croquettes. Sauté salsify in oil and add broth, leek and yogurt. Cover and cook on a low heat for 5 minutes. Add croquettes and cook for another 5 minutes. Add chives, mix well and condiment with salt, pepper and vinegar. Note: add dill if you wish.

# Menu # 15

**French bean salad**
**Prickly pear soup**
**Papadzules**

**French bean salad**

1   cup of small French beans
1   carrot
1   stick of celery
½   leek
1   peeled and chopped red tomato
1   green Julienne pepper
1   yellow Julienne pepper
1   sliced onion
½   handful of chopped parsley
2   sprigs of chopped fresh thyme

**Dressing:**

1   tbs. of mustard
4   tbs. of apple vinegar
6   tbs. of olive oil
     Salt and pepper to taste

Soak French beans overnight. The next day cook them with the carrot, celery, leek, and salt in the water used for soaking water. When cooked, drain (keep broth for a soup) and let vegetables cool. Add the remaining ingredients. Mix the ingredients of the dressing and sprinkle with French beans.

**Prickly pear soup**

5   finely diced tender prickly pears
2   finely diced carrots,
½   onion
3   cloves of garlic
3   red tomatoes
2   fried chipotle chilies

1   Fried pasilla chili peppers
3   tbs. of oil
6   cups of vegetable broth, or to taste
1   potato or diluted flour for thickening

Cook prickly pears in a small amount of salted water and strain. Blend red tomato, onion, garlic and condiment the mixture. Add carrot, prickly pears and enough broth to make a soup. Cover and boil on a low heat until carrots are partly cooked. Remove from heat and stand. Sliced the chilies and serve on top of the prickly pears if you wish desired. You may also add fresh cheese.

**Papadzules**

12   tortillas
6    chopped hard-boiled eggs
10   tbs. of ground pumpkin seeds
1    kilo of red tomato
1    small piece of onion
4    tbs. of oil

Epazote and salt to taste

Cook red tomatoes and onion in a small amount of water with the epazote and salt. Dissolve the pumpkin seeds in a small amount of water. Blend red tomatoes and onion, strain and sauté. Bathe tortillas with pumpkin seeds sauce and stuff with egg. Roll into tacos and bathe with the tomato sauce.

# Menu # 16

**String bean and mushroom salad**
**Three-bean soup**
**Huauzontles**

## String bean and mushroom salad
¾   kilo of cooked and diced string beans
¼   kilo of sliced mushrooms
¼   Julienne onions
¼   red Julienne onion
1   chopped jalapeño chili,
1   cup of chopped red tomato,
2   cloves of garlic
Olive oil to taste
Slightly sauté all ingredients.

### Dressing:

1   lime (juice)
1   orange (juice)
½   tsp. of ground cumin
½   tsp. of ground coriander seeds
¼   cup of olive oil
1   crushed clove of garlic
Mix all ingredients and bathe string beans and champignons.

## Three-bean soup
1   kg. of bayo or canario beans soaked for 12 hours
¼   kg. of black beans
¼   kg. of green beans
2   sprigs of coriander stems
2   pieces of avocado
1   hoja santa leaf
1   small onion
3   cloves of garlic
3   tbs. of sunflower oil
    Toasted bread
    Gruyere cheese
    Emmental cheese

Cook the canario beans with all the ingredients. When cooked, blend and sauté in a little oil. Cook black, and green beans separately with the onion and salt and strain. Add the whole black and green beans to the blended mixture and season together for 10 minutes. Serve soup with toasted bread and with the cheese on top.
Note: save the red and green beans broth for another soup.

## Huauzontles
    Several sprigs of huauzontles
3   red tomatoes
3   cloves of garlic
½   small onion
1   boiled pasilla chili peppers
1   pinch of cumin
½   kg. of panela cheese
2   eggs for coating (optional)
    oil as needed
Partly cook huauzontles in a small amount of salted water and drain well. Arrange several sprigs of huauzontles and put a piece of cheese in the middle. Beat the egg whites until reaching a nougat-like consistency and then add the yolks. Coat the sprigs of huauzontles with flour; then dip in the egg and fry in oil. Blend the tomatoes, onion, garlic and chili separately and then sauté the mixture in oil. Serve huauzontles with this sauce.
For coating without using egg: see sauces, dressings, and more…

# Menu # 17

**Spinach salad**
**Stuffed chayotes**
**Walnut and mushroom pâté**

### Spinach salad
| | |
|---|---|
| 3 | handfuls of fresh spinach |
| 4 | cooked and sliced potatoes |
| 4 | tbs. of chopped chives, |
| 1 | cup of garlic croutons |
| | (See croutons recipe) |

Wash and disinfect spinach; dry the leaves and place them in a dish with the chives; sprinkle with dressing and garnish with croutons.

### Dressing:
| | |
|---|---|
| 1 | tbs. of Dijon mustard |
| 1 | tbs. of chopped red onion |
| ½ | cup of olive oil |
| 1 | lime (juice) or to taste |
| | Sea salt and pepper to taste |

Blend onion, mustard, lime, salt and pepper. Add oil slowly, stirring all the time with hand beater.

### Walnut and mushroom pate
300 grams of mushrooms, finely chopped
100 grams peeled walnut, finely chopped
1 ½ onion, finely chopped
1 garlic clove, smashed and chopped
Olive oil as necessary
Sea salt to taste

Sauté garlic and onion; add mushrooms, and cook for 15 minutes at low heat. Add walnut

### Stuffed chayotes
| | |
|---|---|
| 4 | whole, cooked chayotes |
| 3 | chopped red tomatoes, |
| ½ | large chopped onion |
| 1 | crushed and chopped clove of garlic |
| 2 | chopped red peppers |
| 300 | grams of Panela cheese |
| 4 | tbs. of olive oil |

Sea salt to taste

Cut chayotes in half halves alongside and use a spoon to remove part of the pulp, which is then chopped and mixed with the other ingredients. Sauté and condiment with salt, then stuff the chayote halves with this mixture. Bathe with Béchamel sauce. (See sauces). Bake if you wish.

# Menu # 18

**Sprout salad**
**Celery soup**
**Rice cake**

## Sprout salad
3    cups of mungo bean sprouts
(called soy sprouts)
1½ cups of peeled and chopped red tomatoes
½    cup of chopped onion
3    tbs. of finely chopped coriander
3    tbs. of olive oil
1    diced avocado
1    lime (juice)
Salt or soy sauce to taste
Disinfect and drain sprouts. Mix all ingredients and then add avocado sprinkled with lime juice.

## Parsley dressing:
1    sprig of parsley
¼    cup of oil
1/8    cup of lime juice
3    cloves of garlic
Soy sauce to taste
Seasoning with soy sauce to taste
Blend all ingredients until well mixed.

## Celery soup
6    cups of vegetable broth
4    cups of chopped celery
2    cups of celery juice
1    tsp. of chopped garlic
3    tbs. of chopped onion
4    tbs. of oil
6    tbs. of whole meal
Brown the flour and dilute in the broth. Fry the garlic and onion, add flour and broth, and simmer on a low heat, stirring constantly to prevent lumps forming.
Add celery and its juice. Cook for 3 minutes.

## Rice cake
3    cups of cooked brown rice
5    poblano peppers, grilled and washed,
     cut into slices
4    grilled red tomatoes
½    onion
2    cloves of garlic
2    cups of yogurt or to taste
200 grams of Chihuahua cheese to taste
3    tbs. of oil
     Sea salt to taste
Blend red tomato, onion, and garlic; strain and sauté in oil. Add the strips of chili and season for 5 minutes. Place layers of rice, the chili sauce, cheese and yogurt in a greases dish. Top with cheese. Bake until it melts. Serve hot.

## How to cook whole grain rice
1    cup of brown rice
2    cloves of garlic
½    chopped or Julienne onion
1    stick celery
1    sprig of chopped parsley
3    cups of water or broth
Sea salt to taste
Wash rice well, boil for 3 minutes, rinse with cold water and strain. Sauté the onion and garlic in a little, add water, parsley and rice. Cover and cook on very low heat.
Note: for white rice, leave out parsley.

# Menu # 19

**Purslane salad**
**Energy-giving stew**
**Strawberries with yogurt**

**Purslane salad**
2    cups of washed and chopped purslane
½    cup of finely chopped cabbage
2    cups of diced pineapple
1    cup of diced jícama
1    cup of cooked peas
1    cup of natural yogurt
     Sea salt and pepper to taste
Mix vegetables and fruit. Blend peas with yogurt thoroughly and condiment with salt and pepper. Bathe mixture with this sauce.

**Strawberries with yogurt**
½    kilo of strawberries, smashed
1    cup of natural yogurt
Wash and disinfect strawberries with stem (to avoid smashing); remove stem. Then mix strawberries and yogurt

**Energy-giving stew**
1½   cups of cooked lentils
1½   cups of cooked chickpeas
2    cups of cooked brown rice
1    diced bell pepper
1    diced onion
5    crushed and chopped cloves of garlic
⅛    liter of olive oil
1    pinch of cumin
Aromatic herbs to taste
(bay leaf, thyme and marjoram)
Sea salt to taste

Soak legumes overnight. Cook lentils and legumes separately with aromatic herbs and salt and drain. Cook rice in the broth water used for cooking the lentils and chickpeas. Sauté garlic, onion and pepper, add cumin and lentil, rice and garbanzo, stir, remove from heat and stand. Serve hot. Serve with a sauce of your choice, if you wish.

# Menu # 20

**Raw cauliflower salad**
**Tortilla soup**
**Poblano pepper strips with corn and Mexican squash**

### Raw cauliflower salad
1   small compact, white cauliflower,
2   finely chopped red tomatoes
1   finely chopped onion
3   tbs. of finely chopped parsley,
3   tbs. of finely chopped coriander,
1   diced avocado
    Romaine lettuce leaves
    Sliced radishes to taste
    Olives to taste

Disinfect vegetables and drain. Finely chop cauliflower with its stem. Mix ingredients and sprinkle with dressing. Place a portion of the vegetables in each lettuce leaf and garnish with radishes and olives.

### Dressing:
3   tbs. of mustard
⅔   cup of yogurt
½   cup of mayonnaise
    Salt to taste
    Blend

### Tortilla soup
12   cold, dry and sliced tortillas
4    grill and blended red tomatoes
4    chopped cloves of garlic
½    chopped onion
1    sprig of epazote
4    cups of vegetable broth or water

Oil for frying as needed

Fry the tortillas and remove drain the excess oil with paper towels Sauté garlic, onion and tomato, add the broth, epazote and salt. Let season for 10 minutes on a low heat. Add tortilla and cheese to serve. If you wish, serve with your favorite fried and fired chili.

### Poblano pepper strips with corn and Mexican squash
4   cups of kernel corn
6poblano peppers
4 or 5 chopped Mexican squash
1sliced onion
½   liter of water
250 grams of fresh cheese broken into pieces
5   tbs. of olive oil
Salt to taste

Cook corn in a little oil and water until consumed. Grill peppers, remove veins, wash and cut into strips. Then add to corn with the rest of the oil, onion, Mexican squash and salt. Serve with fresh cheese.

# Menu # 21

**Tricolor salad**
**Chard soup**
**Vegetarian hash**

**Tricolor salad**

1    small lettuce split with the hands
2    thinly sliced red tomatoes
2    thinly sliced avocados
2    thinly sliced sticks of celery
½    Julienne onions
1    grated carrot,
1    grated Mexican squash
2    cooked and sliced beetroots

Disinfect vegetables. Arrange nicely in a dish. Sprinkle with dressing and serve.

**Dressing:**

3    tbs. of soy sauce or to taste
7    tbs. of olive oil or to taste
3    tbs. of lime juice or vinegar
2    crushed and chopped cloves of garlic
     Salt as needed

Mix ingredients and let them stand for at least an hour.

**Chard soup**

8    cups of vegetables broth or water
½    cup of wheat cream (cremola)
½    cup of chopped leek
2    sprigs of chard
2    tbs. of chopped onion
1    tbs. of chopped garlic
4    tbs. of oil

Cook leek in water for 15 minutes. Blend raw chard with the broth. Sauté the wheat cream, garlic and onion in oil and then add the remaining ingredients. Season on a low heat for 10 minutes.

**Vegetarian hash**

2 cups of chopped vegetable meat (wheat gluten)
3    peeled and chopped red tomatoes
1 chopped onion
3 chopped cloves of garlic
2 chopped carrots
20    peeled and chopped almonds
50    grams of seedless raisins
    Salt to taste
    Olive oil

Sauté the garlic and onion add vegetable meat and stir constantly. Add remaining ingredients and condiment with salt. Cover and cook on a low heat for 15 minutes and then leave to stand. Add broth if necessary.

# Menu # 22

**Mineralizing salad**
**Cream of cauliflower**
**Rice fritters**

### Mineralizing salad

| | |
|---|---|
| 1 | small chopped cucumber |
| ½ | cup of chopped celery |
| ½ | cup of chopped lettuce |
| ½ | grated beetroot |
| 1 | grated carrot |
| 6 | sprigs of watercress |
| 2 | sliced radishes |
| 2 | tbs. of grated coconut |

Chinese parsley to taste
Olive oil to taste
Lime juice to taste

Disinfect vegetables. Arrange nicely in a dish. Sprinkle with coconut (or with any oleaginous food), olive oil and lime. Garnish with Chinese parsley and watercress.

### Cream of cauliflower

| | |
|---|---|
| 1 | compact and fresh medium-size cauliflower |
| 1 | sliced onion |
| ½ | leek |
| 2 | cloves of garlic |
| 1 | pinch of anis |
| 3 | tbs. of olive oil |
| 6 | cups of water or as needed |
| | Oregano to taste |
| | Sea salt and pepper to taste |

Cook cauliflower, leek, garlic and anis in water and then blend. Sauté onion and add cauliflower. Condiment with oregano, salt and pepper.

### Rice fritters

| | |
|---|---|
| 1 cup | of cooked brown rice |
| ½ | cup of whole meal flour |
| ½ | cup of chickpea flour |
| ¼ | tsp. of chili powder |
| ¾ | cup of milk or as needed |
| 3 | finely chopped onions |
| 2 | grated carrots |
| ½ | finely chopped red pepper |
| 1 cup | of cottage cheese or yogurt |
| | Mint to taste |
| | Sea salt to taste |
| | Vegetal oil for frying |

Sift dry ingredients. Mix all ingredients. Spoon portions of the mixture on to hot oil. Fry both sides until brown. Drain on a paper towel. Serve with cottage cheese or yogurt and condiment with mint or peppermint.

# Menu # 23

**Wheat salad (tabule)**
**Mexican Squash soup**
**Wild mushrooms in white sauce**
**Wheat cookies**

### Wheat salad (tabule)

1    cup of crashed wheat, soaked for one hour and drained
2    chopped red tomatoes
½    finely chopped large onion
4    tbs. of chopped mint
4    tbs. of finely chopped parsley
½    chopped cucumber
6    lettuce leaves or to taste
½    lime (juice)
4    tbs. of olive oil

Disinfect herbs and lettuce. Mix all ingredients and let stand rest. Place lettuce leaves in a dish and place tabule on each.

### Mexican Squash soup

½    kg. of Mexican squash
½    cup of chopped leek
2    chopped cloves of garlic
1    tbs. of chopped celery
4    tbs. of chopped onion
1    tbs. of oats
6    cups of water
3    tbs. of vegetable oil

Cut and cook the Mexican squash and the leek in water, remove from heat and add oats. Blend when cool. Sauté remaining ingredients and add Mexican squash. Let season for 10 minutes on a low heat. Cover and stand.

### Wild mushrooms in white sauce

1    kilo of wild mushrooms
½    kilo of peas
2    cloves of garlic

Cook peas in a little water. Sauté mushrooms with garlic. Place mushrooms in a dish and bathe with white sauce (see sauces). Garnish with peas.

### Wheat cookies (optional)

2    cups of whole meal flour
2    cups of white flour
1    cup of wheat germ
1    cup of brown sugar
5    tsp. of baking powder
½    cup of yogurt or cold water
1    cup of oil
     Cinnamon or vanilla to taste, optional

Sift dry ingredients well; add yogurt and oil. Spread dough with a rolling pin until to a thickness of ½ cm. Cut with a cookie cutter or a glass. Grease a flat baking tray and place the cookies on it a reasonable distance apart. Bake for 20-30 minutes at a low heat.

# Menu # 24

**Cabbage salad**
**Lentil soup**
**Carrot croquettes**

### Cabbage salad
½    thinly sliced cabbage
¼    red Julienne onion
1    grated carrot
Chopped parsley to taste
Tofu sauce
Disinfect vegetables. Drain well and mix. Season with tofu sauce.
Tofu sauce: tofu, ½ lime; garlic; mustard; sugar; salt and water (all to taste). Blend ingredients.

### Lentil soup
2    cups of lentils soaked for 12 hours
¼    cup of chopped onion
1    cup of red tomato purée or to taste
Oregano
Sea salt to taste
Cook lentils with a piece of onion, two cloves of garlic, a bay leaf and salt. Sauté chopped onion, add tomato and leave to season. Add cooked lentils and season on a low heat for 15 minutes.
Note: you blend a few lentils if you wish. It can be served with fruit, such as diced pineapple, apple, or sliced macho banana. You can also add a tablespoon of yogurt or thick cream.

### Carrot croquettes
7    grated carrots
3    tbs. of wheat germ
½    cup of garbanzo flour
3    tbs. of chopped parsley
3    tbs. of chopped coriander
     Vegetable broth as needed
     Sea salt and pepper to taste
     Oil for frying
Mix all dry ingredients and add broth to form a paste. Spoon portions into hot oil and fry both sides until brown. Serve with tomato sauce or béchamel sauce.
Note: you may use egg instead of garbanzo flour.

### Béchamel vegetable sauce:
½    liter of soy milk
3    tbs. of whole wheat flour
½    chopped onion
Oil
Nutmeg to taste
Sea salt to taste
Sauté onion at a low heat. Add flour and stir. Increase heat and slowly pour in the soy milk, stirring constantly to prevent lumps forming. Condiment with salt and nutmeg.

# Menu # 25

**Watercress salad**
**Cream of Mexican squash and kombu seaweed**
**Rainbow frittata**

## Watercress salad

| | |
|---|---|
| 2 | cups of chopped watercress |
| ½ | chopped Romaine lettuce |
| 1 | chopped red tomato, |
| ½ | cup of chopped coriander |
| ½ | Julienne onions |
| 1 | diced avocado |

**Dressing:**

| | |
|---|---|
| 2 | cloves of garlic |
| | Olive oil |
| 1 | lime (juice) |

Sea salt to taste
Disinfect vegetables. Mix all ingredients and season with this dressing or any other of you favorites.

## Cream of Mexican squash and kombu seaweed

| | |
|---|---|
| ½ | kg. of sliced Mexican squash |
| ½ | small chopped onion |
| ½ | small chopped leek |
| 6 | cups of water or vegetable broth |
| 100 | grams of almonds |
| 2 | tbs. of olive oil |
| 2 | sheets (pieces) kombu seaweed |
| | Sea salt to taste |

Cook squash and leek in water. Soak almonds in hot water for peeling. Cut the seaweed into small pieces and soak. Blend squash, leek and almonds. Sauté onion, add the blended ingredients and seaweed; boil for 10 minutes. Add a tablespoon of oats to thicken.

## Rainbow frittata

| | |
|---|---|
| 1 | cup of beans soaked overnight |
| 2 | eggs |
| 2 | tbs. of vegetable oil |
| 2 | grated carrots |
| 2 | grated Mexican squash |
| 2 | Julienne onions |
| 3 | cups of kernel corn |
| 2 | tbs. of chopped basil |
| 2 | tbs. of chopped mint |

100 grams of grated Chihuahua cheese
Sea salt and black pepper to taste
Blend beans with eggs until an even mixture is produced. Sauté onion, add carrot and squash (zucchini) and cook for 5 minutes. Then add beans, vegetables, corn, basil and condiment with pepper and salt. Place mixture in a greased dish and bake at a moderate heat for 30 minutes or until brown. Serve with cottage cheese or yogurt with mint or coconut cream with lime or peppermint.

# Menu # 26

**Cucumber and apple salad**
**Olla Mole**
**Apple croquettes**

**Cucumber and apple salad**
1    disinfected Romaine lettuce
2    sliced cucumbers
3    diced apples
1    lime (juice)

Soak apples in a little water with lime for 5 minutes to prevent avoid oxidation and then drain. Soak cucumbers in salted water and drain. Place the lettuce in a dish and add apple and cucumber. Garnish with mayonnaise or any other light dressing.

**Apple croquettes**
1    kilo of golden  apples
2    cups of whole wheat flour
1    cup of white flour
1    cup of wheat germ
1    cup of brown sugar
5    tbs. of baking powder
2    eggs
1    tbs. of warm water or as needed
     Oil as needed for frying

Cut apples into slices after removing the core. Sift flours, baking powder and sugar. Add warm water, eggs and apples. Let stand for ½ hour. Spoon portions of the mixture onto hot oil and fry until brown. Serve with papaya puree, cream or cottage cheese.

**Olla Mole**
3    fried Guajillo chili without veins
1    fried Ancho chili without veins
1    fried Pasilla chili without veins
3    ears of corns cut into pieces
1     cup of string beans, either whole or in halves
1    cup of chopped cabbage
2    cups of squash flower
8    diced  Mexican squash
2    Xoconoxtles (peeled and seedless)
½    kilo of sliced mushrooms
     (or other varieties)
2    finely chopped sprigs of epazote,
3    liters of boiling water
1    large onion
4    cloves of garlic
50 grams of chopped manchego cheese
(may be cut into strips)
¼    kilo of corn dough
2    tbs. of vegetable oil
4    limes
Sea salt to taste

Mix dough with cheese, epazote and salt, make into small balls and make a hole in the middle with your finger. Blend chilies, ½ onion and garlic and then sauté in oil. Add boiling water, corn and all ingredients and  cook at a low heat for 20 minutes.

# Menu # 27

**Soy bean sprout salad**
**Wheat soup**
**Quintonil pie**

### Soy bean sprout salad
4   cups of mungo beans sprouts
1   cup of peeled and chopped red tomato
½   cup of sliced onion
½   cup of chopped parsley and coriander
4   tbs. of grated cheese
4   tbs. of olive oil
     Soy sauce to taste

Wash and disinfect bean sprouts, parsley, and coriander and drain. Mix all ingredients and season with soy sauce, oil and cheese, or you may use your favorite dressing. The soy bean sprouts may be changed for any other, such as wheat, garbanzo, etcetera.

### Wheat soup
½   cup of soaked wheat cream (cremola)
½   cup of thick crushed wheat (soaked)
6   cups of vegetables broth
½   cup of chopped onion
½   cup of chopped red pepper
½   cup of chopped string beans
½   cup of chopped Mexican squash
2   chopped cloves of garlic
1   tbs. of vegetable oil
½   tsp. of marjoram
¼   tsp. of thyme
1   bay leaf
Sea salt to taste

Cook wheat in broth for 10 minutes. Blend half of it with the water used for cooking.

Sauté garlic, onion and pepper, and add broth with wheat and the remaining ingredients. When the mixture comes to the boil, lower the heat and season for 10 minutes.

### Quintonil pie
½   kg. chopped quintonils without the stem
1   finely chopped onion
2   tbs. of oil or vegetarian butter
½   cup of Chihuahua cheese
½   cup of ricotta o cottage cheese
½   cup of grated strong-flavored cheese
4   tbs. of grated Parmesan cheese
4   lightly beaten eggs
¼   tsp. of nutmeg powder
1   pinch of ground pepper
3   tbs. of olive oil
     Salt to taste
¾   of kilo of puff paste
     (Approximately)

Cook quintonils in a little of water for 3-5 minutes. Drain liquid thoroughly and allow to cool. Sauté onion in oil. Mix onion, quintonils and cheeses. Blend eggs with pepper and nutmeg, and then add quintonils. Divide puff paste into two parts. Line a previously greased mold with one part and pour in the quintonil mixture, cover with remaining puff paste, join the edges well and then coat with oil or egg. Bake until brown.
Note: quintonils may be replaced by chard.

# Menu # 28

**Complete salad**
**Corn soup**
**Eggplant with cashews**
**Corn bread**

## Complete salad
3   lettuce leaves
1   finely chopped leek
2   medium-size potatoes, cooked
¼   chopped onion,
1   chopped clove of garlic,
1   washed and grilled red pepper
½   lime (juice)
    Olives to taste
    Virgin olive oil

Finely slice and peeled potatoes; season with oil, lime, onion and garlic, then let stand for 1 hour. Add lettuce in pieces, and leek, olives, mixing thoroughly, before serving the salad. Garnish with strips of pepper.

## Corn soup
2   cups of kernel corn
6   cups of water or vegetable broth
4   tbs. of chopped leek
6   tbs. of chopped celery
1   sprig of mint
2   tbs. of vegetal oil
Sea salt to taste

Cook corn, leek, and celery in the broth. Sauté garlic and onion and then add vegetables with mint and salt; cook for a few minutes.

## Eggplant with Cashews
3   sliced eggplants
3   peeled and chopped red tomatoes
1   grilled, washed and sliced red pepper
5   crushed cloves of garlic
4   tbs. of olive oil
100 grams of cashews
5   tbs. of chopped parsley
    Sea salt to taste
    Oil as necessary

Peel eggplants and slice and soak in hot salted water for 2 hours. Sauté in oil a low heat 3 cloves of garlic and eggplant until brown. Put eggplant in a dish, prepare the sauce and pour on eggplant. Garnish with parsley.

Sauce: Sauté the remaining garlic cloves in 4 tablespoons of olive oil over a low heat, and then add red tomato. Cook lightly, add salt, cashews, and bell pepper. Cook for 5 minutes.

## Corn bread (optional)
3   cups of kernel corn
4   eggs
1½  butter bars, or vegetarian margarine
1   tbs. of baking powder
1   cup of brown sugar
1   cup of whole meal flour

Sift flour and baking powder. Blend remaining ingredients and mix with flour. Pour into a baking pan already greased and covered with flour. Bake at 350ºF for one hour until brown.

# Menu # 29

**Starch salad**
**Cream of avocado**
**Strips of chili with broad beans and Mexican squash**

### Starch salad
3 cups of cooked and diced potatoes or sweet potatoes.
3 diced golden pear-shaped apples
1½ cups of finely chopped celery,
Mayonnaise to taste
Peeled and chopped almonds
Salt to taste
6 disinfected lettuce leaves
Mix celery, potato and apple and then sprinkle with salt. Form a bed of lettuce in a dish, place remaining ingredients on top, bathe with mayonnaise and garnish with almonds or any of your favorite dressings.

### Mayonnaise without eggs:
1 cup of virgin olive oil
⅓ cup of soy milk
½ clove of garlic
½ lime (juice)
 Salt to taste
Blend until perfectly mixed. You can make colored sauces with: cooked carrot (pink), cooked beetroot (pink), avocado (green); mustard (yellow) and fried tomato (red).

### Cream of avocado
5 ripe avocados
6 cups of vegetable broth
7 tbs. of ground goat or fresh cheese
 Sea salt to taste
Blend avocados in a cup of broth and add the remaining broth already seasoned with soy sauce. Serve immediately with cheese on top. This soup is cold.

### Strips of chili with broad beans and Mexican squash
8 grilled, washed and, sliced poblano peppers
2 cups of green broad beans, peeled and cooked in a little water
2 cups of diced Mexican squash
1 sliced onion
250 grams of ground panela cheese or vegetarian cheese.
4 tbs. of oil
Salt to taste
Sauté onion, and remaining ingredients together. Add a little of the water in which the broad beans were cooked, and salt. Boil at a low hat for 10 minutes. Serve with cheese on top.

# Menu # 30

**Ceviche**
**Chickpea stew**
**Corn cake**

## Ceviche

½   finely chopped onion,
2   finely chopped garlic cloves
1   chopped red tomato
2   cups of chopped mushrooms
1   grated Mexican squash
1   grated carrot
3   tbs. of lime juice
Olive oil to taste
Finely chopped coriander to taste
Tomato ketchup to taste
Mix all ingredients and serve.

## Corn cake

6   cups of kernel corn
1   cup of brown sugar
200   grams of butter or vegetarian margarine
6   eggs
1   cup of rice flour
1   pinch of bicarbonate
2   tbs. of baking powder
Thoroughly blend corn raw with brown sugar and egg yolks. Sift flour, bicarbonate and baking powder. Whip egg whites to a nougat consistency. Mix corn, flour and egg whites. Pour mixture in a mold already greased and cover with breadcrumbs. Bake at a moderate heat.

## Chickpea stew

½   kg.  soaked and cooked chickpeas
¼   kg.  sliced mushrooms (optional)
1   grilled, washed, and sliced red pepper
1   large sliced onion
2   crushed cloves of garlic
2   grilled red tomatoes
2   tbs. of chopped parsley
½   tbs. of rosemary
1   pinch of cumin powder
2   tbs. of oil
Salt and pepper to taste
Blend a quarter of chickpeas with a part of cooking water. Sauté the garlic, onion, and pepper. Add tomato, blended and sieved. Add the rest of the broth, the whole blended chickpeas, mushrooms and all other ingredients. Boil slowly until mushrooms are cooked.

# Menu # 31

**Pasta salad**
**French bean soup**
**Asparagus and apples**

## Pasta salad
400 grams of small pasta
½ onion
2tsp. of salt
1tbs. of oil
5peeled and chopped red tomatoes
1tsp. of ground oregano
5tsp. of olive oil
1 diced manchego cheese or vegetarian cheese
 Mayonnaise to taste
 Salt and pepper to taste
Cook pasta in water with onion and salt for 10 minutes, avoiding overcooking. Strain it. Mix remaining ingredients and add to pasta; stir gently.

## French bean soup
1 cup of small cooked French beans
3 grilled red tomatoes
1 chopped medium onion
2 chopped carrots
1 chopped turnip
2 chopped Mexican squash
1 chopped small leek
3 crushed cloves of garlic
8 cups of French bean broth
 Sea salt to taste

Blend tomato and strain. Sauté garlic, onion and vegetables; add tomato and half of the French beans, blend the other part, then strain and add. Simmer for 15 minutes. Serve hot.

## Asparagus and apples
15 asparagus tips cooked *al dente*
½ cup of diced apple
1 chopped clove of garlic
2 tbs. of olive oil
1 pinch of nutmeg
1 pinch of cinnamon powder
 Salt and white pepper to taste
Sauté garlic, asparagus, and apple together with condiments for 3 minutes

# Menu # 32

**Italian salad**
**Spaghetti with Ragu Sauce**
**Green *mole***

**Italian salad**
2      peeled and chopped red tomatoes
½      chopped onion
2      chopped sticks of celery
1      handful of chopped spinach,
¼      cup of finely chopped cabbage
½      chopped French lettuce

**Dressing:**
3      tbs. of orange juice
3      tbs. of lime juice
3      tbs. of grapefruit juice
6      tbs. of olive oil
¼      tsp of oregano
Mix ingredients and sprinkle with dressing before serving.

**Pasta with Ragu Sauce**
1      packet of cooked spaghetti

**Ragu sauce:**
4      tbs. of olive oil
1      cup of finely chopped carrot
½      cup of finely chopped onion
1      cup of finely chopped celery
1      cup of finely chopped mushrooms
3      cups of red tomato paste
     Vegetables broth as needed
     Soy milk to taste
     Sea salt to taste
Sauté vegetables and then add remaining ingredients; simmer for one hour. Serve on top of spaghetti.

**Green mole**
10      lettuce leaves
8      radish leaves
½      cup of coriander
½      cup of parsley
4      sprigs of epazote
1      sprig of mint
1      large onion
1      cup of pumpkin seeds
4      cloves of garlic
     Green chilies to taste
½      kg. textured soy (prepared)
2tbs. of vegetable oil
Blend all ingredients, except soy, and season in oil. Cook on a low heat for 15 minutes.

**How to prepare soy:**
Place all aromatic herbs and the ones in your pantry in water. When they have released their flavor, remove them and add textured soy until hydrated, or boil for 5 minutes. Drain well. Sauté in oil. Ready for any dish.

# Menu # 33

**American salad**
**Tofu and walnut hamburger**
**Apple soufflé**

## American salad
1    cup of cooked rice
1    cup of finely chopped celery
1    cup of chopped bell pepper
4    chopped apples
**Dressing:**
1    cup of yogurt
4    tbs. of olive oil (optional)
1    tbs. of mustard
2    tsp. of red paprika
    Salt and pepper to taste
Soak apples in water with lime for 10 minutes to avoid oxidation. Mix ingredients and season with dressing. Garnish with chopped parsley if you wish.

## Apple soufflé
1    kg. of sliced apples
1½    cups of brown sugar, or to taste
4    eggs
1    egg white
4    tbs. of butter or vegetarian margarine
Vanilla and cinnamon to taste
Cook apples in butter on a low heat; add sugar, vanilla and cinnamon. Mash into a puree, allow to cool, and add yolks and egg whites gently beaten to a nougat-like consistency. Pour in previously greased mold. Bake 25 minutes at a moderate heat. Serve immediately with milk cream or yoghurt.

## Tofu and walnut hamburger
6    whole grain buns
6    lettuce leaves
6    slices of cooked beetroot
¼    cup of yogurt

## Hamburgers
1    cup of tofu (soy cheese)
½    cup of chickpea flour
2    grated carrots
2    grated Mexican squash
¼    cup of finely chopped walnut
1    cup of breadcrumbs
2    tsp. of chopped coriander
2    crushed cloves of garlic with sea salt
2    tbs. of Dijon mustard
3    tbs. of sesame seeds
3    tbs. of vegetable oil
    Salt and pepper to taste
Mix all hamburger ingredients, except sesame seeds. Make 6 hamburger patties and pass them over the seeds. Fry until brown. Cut rolls in half and cover with lettuce, hamburger, beetroot (optional) and a spoonful of yogurt. Serve immediately.
Note: add onion if you wish.

# Menu # 34

**Nicoise salad**
**Pearl barley soup**
**Eggplant** *au gratin*

**Nicoise salad**
1    lettuce cut into pieces
3    cooked and diced potatoes
250 grams of cooked and diced green beans
3    chopped red tomatoes
10   olives
2    tbs. of olive oil
1    tbs. of apple vinegar
½    tbs. of mustard
Salt and pepper to taste
Mix all ingredients well. Add more dressing if needed.

**Pearl barley soup**
6    tbs. of pearl barley (one per person)
2    grated carrots
2    grated Mexican squash
1    grated turnip
1    chopped bell pepper
½    chopped onion
2    chopped cloves of garlic
2    chopped sticks of celery
1    sprig of mint or to taste
8    cups of water or as needed
     Sea salt to taste
Cook barley in water for 25 minutes. Sauté garlic, onion and pepper and add remaining ingredients. Then add this mixture to the barley and season for another 5 minutes.

**Eggplant** *au gratin*
2    eggplants
2    large red tomatoes
½    onion
3    cloves of garlic
1    cup of water or as needed
100  grams of grated Chihuahua cheese
100  grams of grated panela cheese
Oregano to taste
 Sea salt to taste
Slice eggplants and soak in salted water for ½ hour to prevent oxidation. Blend red tomato, onion, garlic and sauté. Add water, oregano and salt. Place layers of eggplant in a dish and bathe with the sautéed tomato mixture and cheese. Add cheeses and bake for 10-15 minutes.

# Menu # 35

**Apple salad**
**Mushroom soup**
**Rajas and cheese tamales**

### Apple salad
6   finely diced golden pear-shaped apples
1   cup of finely chopped pineapple
1   cup of finely chopped celery
½   cup of finely chopped carrot
1   cup of chopped walnut
½   cup of raisins
½   cup of pine nuts
1½ cup of thick yogurt
½   cup of mayonnaise
1   tsp. of brown sugar

Blend yogurt, mayonnaise and sugar. Add celery, apple and pineapple. Add remaining ingredients to serve.

### Mushroom soup
400   grams of chopped mushrooms
1½   cup of soy milk
3cups of water or as needed
2chopped medium-size onions
2tbs. of soy oil
1tsp. of sesame seed oil
  Sea salt and pepper to taste
Slightly sauté onion in both oils. Add remaining ingredients, cook on a low heat for 15 minutes. Serve hot.

### Rajas and cheese tamales
2   kilos of corn flour
1½   cups of corn oil
1   clove of garlic
½   onion
Green tomato peel water as needed
Salt to taste
1   handful of soaked corn leaves
Stew of poblano peppers slices with onion, red tomato and fresh cheese
To prepare green tomato peel water: Boil water with green tomato peel until ready.
In a bit of water blend onion and garlic. Mix corn flour, oil, salt, onion, garlic and green tomato water; beat until "eyes" are formed. Place a spoonful of dough and a little of the poblano-strip stew in each of the corn leaves. Steam the tamales or cook in a bain-marie. To make sweet tamales, use a sweet filling of your choice instead of salt, use sugar.

# Menu # 36

**Mexican squash salad**
**Lentil soup**
**Spring casserole**

### Mexican squash salad
3  cups of grated Mexican squash
1½  cups pf chopped red tomato
½  finely chopped onion
½  cup of chopped coriander (cilantro)
Mix all these ingredients.

### Dressing:
3  peeled avocados without the bone
3  cloves of garlic
1  cup of yogurt
1  tbs. of grill sesame seeds
1  tbs. of olive oil
Soy sauce to taste
White pepper to taste
Soy milk as needed
Blend all ingredients thoroughly, except sesame seeds that are used to garnish.

### Lentil soup
1  cup of lentils soaked for 12 hours
8  cups of water
½  sliced leek
3  chopped cloves of garlic
½  small finely chopped onion
1  cold toasted roll cut into squares
Oregano to taste
Sea salt to taste
Cook lentils with leek, blend and strain. Sauté garlic and onion and add lentils with their broth. Cook at a low heat for 10 minutes. Add oregano and serve with pieces of toasted bread.

Note: you may replace lentils with chickpeas, beans, broad beans, rice, and etcetera.

### Spring casserole
1  cup of sliced potato
1  cup of broccoli cut in pieces
1  cup of finely chopped celery
1  cup of sliced onion
1  cup of diced Mexican squash
1  cup of grated cabbage
½  cup of chopped parsley
½  cup of vegetable broth
½  cup of fresh or Manchego cheese or vegetarian cheese.
3  sliced red tomatoes
3  chopped cloves of garlic
2  tbs. of thyme
1  tsp. of rosemary
Sea salt and pepper to taste
Place the vegetables in a dish in the following order: potatoes, broccoli, celery, onion, squash, cabbage, and tomato. Mix broth with herbs and bathe vegetables with it; top with cheese. Cover the baking pan (glass pan) with aluminum foil and bake at 180ºC for 15 minutes.

# Menu # 37

**String bean salad**
**Rice Mexican style**
**Purslane in green sauce**

**String bean salad**
2    cups of string beans cooked *al dente*
and cut into pieces
1    small sliced onion
2    peeled and diced red tomatoes
1    sliced bell pepper
⅛    cup of olive oil
½    tsp. of oregano
1    lime (juice)
Salt and pepper to taste
Mix all ingredients together.

**Rice Mexican style**
1½    cups of whole grain rice
1    cup of peeled English peas
¾    cup of diced carrots
¾    cup of chopped parsley
½    cup of chopped coriander (cilantro)
½    onion
4    cloves of garlic
2    red tomatoes
2    sliced cuaresmenos chilies
4 tbs. of vegetable oil
6 cups of water
Salt to taste

Wash rice, boil in water for 3 minutes, rinse with cold water and strain; sauté until light brown and add formerly blended and the red tomato blended with garlic and onion. Add carrots, peas, cilantro, and water. Cover and simmer for 45 minutes. When it has softened and dried, add parsley and chilies. Cook for another 3 minutes an turn out the heat.

**Purslane in green sauce**
1    kg. of purslane
½    kilo of green tomato
½    cup of coriander (cilantro)
1    sprig of epazote
½    onion
3    diced Mexican squash
3    cloves of garlic
3    tbs. of vegetable oil
Green chilies to taste
Sea salt to taste
Wash purslane and washed until only the tender stems and leaves remain. Cook in a little water. Blend all remaining ingredients to prepare the sauce. Fry until well seasoned. Add purslane with the water in which it was cooked and cook for another 10 minutes.
**Note:** add all herbs you have handy if you wish.

# Menu # 38

**Broad-bean salad**
**Vegetable pastries**
**Garden-style cabbage**

## Broad-bean salad

1    cup of cooked fresh broad beans
1    lettuce split by hand
1    cup of alfalfa bean sprouts
2    grated carrots
2    sticks stems of finely chopped celery
½    cup of chopped cabbage or cauliflower
2    tbs. of sesame seeds
1    tbs. of sunflower seeds
Mix all the ingredients.

## Dressing:

Mix 2 parts lime juice to 1 part olive or peanut oil. Add onion, garlic, ground dry herbs and salt to taste. Mix all ingredients, and season.

## Vegetable pastries

200    grams of chopped mushrooms
1 finely chopped onion
2        handfuls of chopped spinach
  Cumin to taste
  Sea salt to taste
  Oil as needed for frying
Mix all the ingredients.

## Dough:

¼    kilo of whole meal flour
¼    kilo of white flour
¼    kilo of chickpea flour
1 tsp. of baking soda
½    tsp. of brown sugar
  Salt and water as needed

Blend the ingredients thoroughly. Roll the dough, cut into circles (with a glass), and then stuff with vegetables, fold, moisten edges borders and press with a fork to seal the closing pastries correctly. You can bake or fry them.

## Garden-style cabbage

1    thinly sliced medium-size cabbage
¾    finely chopped onion
3    peeled and chopped red tomatoes
1    tbs. of apple vinegar
1    tsp. of brown sugar
½    tsp of peeled and grated ginger root
3    tbs. of olive oil
Sea salt to taste
1    Stale roll (torta bread)
Sauté onion in oil, add cabbage and keep cooking. Add remaining ingredients except the bread; mix and fry together. Place the bread on the cabbage (to prevent gas and unpleasant smells); cover the pot without adding water and cook on a low heat for 10 minutes. Remove the bread and throw it away. If you wish to cook *au gratin*, pour place the cabbage in a dish and cover with cheese to taste and then bake at a moderate heat until melted.

# Menu # 39

**Eggplant salad**
**Mexican squash soup**
**Chickpea gorditas**

## Eggplant salad
5    small eggplants
3    peeled and sliced red tomatoes
4    tbs. of fresh chopped basil
     Recently grounded black pepper
**Dressing:**
4    tbs. of olive oil
2    tbs. of apple vinegar
2    crushed gloves of garlic

Cut eggplants into lengths 1 cm wide, coat with plenty of olive oil and fry on a frying plate until tender. Mix dressing and let stand. Place the hot eggplant slices in a dish, cover with tomato and sprinkle with basil, pepper and dressing. Repeat layers until you have finished. Cover dish with tin foil and refrigerate overnight or for at least 10-12 hours. Serve with Arabian bread and yogurt. Serve as an entrée or take it on a picnic.

## Mexican squash soup
6    cups of water or vegetable broth
½    kg. Mexican squash
½    cup of sliced leek
2    tbs. of whole oats
2    chopped cloves of garlic
¼    finely chopped onion
1    finely chopped sticks of celery
2    tbs. of oil

Cook leek and Mexican squash in water at a low heat flame until they are *al dente*. Remove from heat, add oats and stand until cold. Blend squash, leek and oats. Sauté the garlic, onion and celery, add squash and season for 10 minutes.

## Chickpea gorditas
¼    kg. corn dough
¼    kg. chickpeas, cooked and blended
¼    onion
2    grated carrots
100  grams of grated Chihuahua cheese or vegetarian cheese
Sea salt to taste

Blend chickpeas with onion, add remaining ingredients and prepare the gorditas. Cook on a frying plate. Serve with your favorite chili sauce.

**Note:** you may add diverse vegetables to taste, oregano, ground coriander seeds, parsley, mushrooms, cheese, etcetera.

# Menu # 40

**Okara ceviche**
**Corn soup**
**Tamales a la Provencal**

## Okara ceviche

1½ cups of okara
1 cup of peeled and chopped red tomatoes
1 cup of chopped mushrooms
½ cup of chopped olives
1 cup of diced avocado
  cup of finely chopped green chilies or
    to taste
3 tbs. of finely chopped coriander
  Soaked fungus or hijiki seaweed,
    amount to taste
  Lime juice to taste
  Tomato ketchup to taste (see sauces)
  Limes cut into four
  Habanera-style whole meal cookies

Mix ingredients, place them in the center of a dish and marinate with tomato ketchup. Garnish with cookies and lime around the edge of the dish.

## Corn soup

3 cups of kernel corn
6 cups of water or as necessary
½ thinly sliced leek
6 sprigs of chopped fresh watercress
1 sprig of mint
2 tbs. of vegetable oil
  Sea salt to taste

Blend corn with a little water, strain and pour the rest into boiling water. Sauté leek, add corn, mint, and salt. Season it at a low heat for 15 minutes. Serve hot. Garnish with watercress.

## Tamales a la Provenzal

500 grams of chopped mushrooms
10 finely chopped cloves of garlic
1sprig of parsley
 Olive oil to taste
 Salt to taste

Sauté garlic in oil, add mushrooms, parsley and salt.

## Dough:

1 kilo of flour for tamales
¾ cup of vegetable oil or as needed
1 bundle of soaked corn leaves
1 heaped tbs. of baking powder
Water as needed
 Sea salt to taste

Sieve flour and baking powder; add oil and about 2 cups of water or the amount needed to form firm dough, not limp. Place a spoonful of dough and stuffing on each leaf. Close the leaf and steam or cook bain-marie. If you want to use a stuffing instead of mushrooms, use squash flower, Mexican squash, grains of ears of corn and strips of poblano pepper.

# Menu # 41

**Cauliflower salad**
**Potato and scallion soup**
**Mexican squash a la crème**
**Potato croquettes**

**Cauliflower salad**

1   tender compact and white cauliflower
1   large sliced onion
1   tsp. of oregano powder
5   tbs. of olive oil
3   tbs. of lime juice
150 grams of Panela cheese or
Vegetarian cheese
Soy sauce or salt to taste

Soak onion in lime juice. Cut half of the cauliflower into small pieces; cook the other half and let cool. Cut into small pieces. Mix ingredients and garnish with cheese.

**Potato and leek soup**

¾   of kilo of potatoes
1   sliced leek
4   tbs. of finely chopped onion
1   finely chopped clove of garlic
1   tbs. of vegetable oil
Disinfected parsley to taste
Sea salt to taste

Cook potato and leek together; allow to cool and blend. Sauté garlic and onion in the oil, mix both ingredients and simmer for 10 minutes. Serve with chopped parsley.
Note: potato may be sliced, not blended.

**Mexican squash a la crème**

6   sliced Mexican squash
     Aromatic herbs to taste
1   cup of natural yogurt or thick cream
¼   finely chopped onion
2   finely chopped cloves of garlic
     Salt to taste
     Oil as necessary

Cook the squash *al dente* with a little water and the herbs. Sauté garlic and onion and then add cream. Place squash in a dish and bathe with cream.
Note: you may place put cheese on top and cook *au gratin* in the oven.

**Potato croquettes**

3   cups of cooked potato puree
½   cup of chopped parsley
2   eggs
½   tsp. of cumin powder
     Salt and pepper to taste
     Breadcrumbs as needed
     Vegetable oil as needed for frying

Mix potato puree with egg yolks, parsley, cumin, salt and pepper. Add egg whites beaten to a nougat-like consistency. Shape the croquettes, dip in the breadcrumbs and fry. Place in serving dish and garnish with chopped lettuce.
**Note:** you may replace eggs with garbanzo flour.

# Menu # 42

**Rice salad**
**Garlic soup**
**Chard soufflé**

## Rice salad

1   cup of cooked whole grain rice (or
     that left over from the day before)
½   cup of lentil bean sprouts
1   cup of peeled and chopped red tomatoes
½   cup of red tomato juice
½   cup of finely chopped celery
1   cup of finely chopped lettuce
100 grams of diced Panela cheese or
Vegetarian cheese
Mix all ingredients and bathe you're your
favorite dressing (see dressings).

## Garlic soup

6   cups of hot vegetable broth
1   large garlic bulb
3   tbs. of vegetable oil
4   lightly beaten eggs
1   lime (juice)
1   whole meal bread, diced and toasted
Cook garlic bulb in broth. Blend and strain.
Fry 5 cloves of finely chopped garlic in oil, add
garlic broth and boil for 10 minutes; remove
from heat, add egg with salt and stir well.
Serve with drops of lime and toasted bread.

## Chard soufflé

600  grams of chard
1cup of white sauce
3eggs
 Nutmeg to taste
 Sea salt to taste
Cook chard in 4 spoonfuls of water; drain well
and make into a puree. Mix with white sauce
and egg yolks and condiment with nutmeg
and salt. Add egg whites slowly beaten to a
nougat-like consistency. Pour in a dish and
bake for 20 minutes. Serve immediately.

## White sauce

1   tbs. of butter or vegetarian margarine
1   tbs. of corn flour or wheat flour
¼   tbs. of mustard powder
1   tbs. of cream or natural yogurt
½   liter of milk or soy milk
     Salt and pepper to taste
Blend milk, cream, corn flour, mustard, salt
and pepper. Melt butter and pour mixture
on it. Simmer and stir constantly to prevent
lumps forming. If too thick, add milk.

# Menu # 43

**Mixed salad**
**Tortilla soup**
**Poblano peppers stuffed with beans and cheese**

## Mixed salad

- Cooked peas
- Cooked string beans
- Grated Mexican squash
- Grated carrots
- Grated beetroots
- Lettuce
- Sliced red tomato
- Julienne onion

Quantities to taste. Mix all ingredients and sprinkle with lime or apple vinegar, olive oil, salt and oregano; you may use another of you favorite dressings.

## Tortilla soup

10    tortillas
3     blended red tomatoes
¼     finely chopped onion
2     finely chopped cloves of garlic
1     sprig of epazote
6     cups of water
100   grams of grated cheese

Cut tortillas into strips and fry until brown; remove the oil with a paper towel. Sauté garlic, onion, and tomato add water and epazote. Let season for a few minutes. Add tortilla and garnish with cheese to serve. You may serve with fried slices of Pasilla chili.

## Poblano peppers stuffed with beans and cheese

6     grill and washed poblano peppers
1     cup of beans, cooked and blended
½     finely chopped onion
2     finely chopped of cloves of garlic
100   grams of grated Chihuahua cheese or vegetarian cheese
100   grams of grated Panela cheese or
2     tbs. of vegetable oil

Fry garlic, onion and beans in oil. Stuff the chilies with fried beans and cheese.

## Sauce:

4     dry-fried red tomatoes
½     onion
3     cloves of garlic
2     tbs. of vegetable oil

Blend tomato, onion and garlic, then strain, sauté in oil and condiment with salt. Bathe the chilies in this sauce. Another option is to serve with guacamole and cabbage.

# Menu # 44

**Pineapple and apple salad**
**Carrot soup**
**Eggplant with wheat**

### Pineapple and apple salad
3    diced apples
1    small diced pineapple
1    natural yogurt
1    tbs. of mayonnaise
¼    tbs. of mustard
     Walnuts to taste
     Salt to taste
Mix all the ingredients.

### Carrot soup
6    carrots
1    medium-size potato
½    leek
5    cups of water
     Chopped parsley to taste
Wash carrots, potato and leek well. Slice them and boil in water and simmer until half cooked. Add salt, wait until warm and blend. Boil a little more and serve. Garnish with parsley.

### Eggplant with wheat
4    medium-size eggplants
2    chopped red tomatoes
1    chopped onion
3    cloves of garlic
2    chopped green chilies
1    cup of thick wheat, soaked and drained
½    cup of cooked chickpeas
2    pinches of cinnamon powder
     Chopped parsley to taste
     Chopped mint to taste
Sea salt to taste
Wash eggplants, cut in half long ways, scoop out flesh with a spoon and place everything in cold salted water for ½ hour. Sauté garlic, onion, green chili, tomato, wheat, chickpeas, eggplant pulp, salt, and cinnamon. Let season on a low heat for 10 minutes. Add parsley and mint and remove from heat. Stuff eggplants with this mixture. Place on a flat pan and pour on sauce. Let season on a low heat for 15 minutes.

### Sauce:
4    grill red tomatoes
½    small onion
3    cloves of garlic
Blend ingredients and strain. Let season in 2 spoonfuls of oil for 10 minutes.

# Menu # 45

**Mixed salad**
**Summer artichokes**
**Chickpea puree**

### Mixed salad

1   cup of sliced Cos lettuce
1   cup of sliced red lettuce
1   cup of sliced Romaine lettuce
3   red tomatoes cut into four
1   stick of celery, chopped
1   sliced cucumber
1   grated carrot
1   grated or diced jícama

Mix lettuces, carrot, jícama and celery; garnish with tomato and cucumber. Add your favorite dressing (see dressings).

### Summer artichokes

7    cooked artichokes,
½    finely chopped onion
4    chopped hard-boiled eggs
100  grams of Parmesan cheese
1    cup of French dressing or mustard

Mix onion, eggs and cheese. Place artichokes in a dish; open the leaves and bathe with the above mixture. Sprinkle with dressing (see dressings). Serve cold.

### Chickpea puree (humus)

2    cups of cooked garbanzo
4    tbs of sesame paste (tahini)
3    limes (juice)
3    cloves of garlic
15   walnuts (in halves) or to taste
     Walnuts to garnish
     Salt to taste
     Olive oil to taste
     Paprika to taste
     Chinese parsley to garnish

Blend chickpeas, sesame seed paste, lime juice, garlic, salt, and walnuts with a little of the water in which the chickpeas were cooked. Place in a dish and garnish with paprika, olive oil, walnuts and Chinese parsley. Serve with Arabian bread cut into triangles.

# Menu # 46

**Pansanela salad**
**Vegetable and pine nut tortellini**
**Stuffed and grilled potatoes**

**Pansanela salad**
3    diced red tomatoes
10   chopped olives
½    sliced onion
1    finely chopped clove of garlic
3    sprigs of basil finely chopped
1    bread roll diced and toasted
2    tbs. of apple vinegar
4    tbs. of olive oil
     Sea salt to taste
Mix all the ingredients.

**Vegetable and pine nut tortellini**
500   grams of spinach-stuffed tortellini
¼     cup of pine nuts
¼     cup of diced carrots
¼     cup of diced turnip
¼     cup of diced green pepper
¼     cup of diced red pepper
1 cup of vegetable broth or as needed
2 crushed and chopped cloves of garlic
3 tbs. of olive oil
 Basil finely crushed
 Sea salt and pepper to taste
Boil vegetables for 2 minutes in salted water
and drain. Cook pasta *al dente*. Sauté garlic,
vegetables, and pine nuts in oil until brown.
Add broth and condiment with salt and
pepper. Bring to the boil and add tortellini.
Blend and allow to heat. Garnish with basil.

**Stuffed and grilled potatoes**
6       medium-size potatoes
2       tbs. of butter or vegetarian margarine
½       finely chopped onion
250     grams of mushrooms
2 cups of white sauce
        Parmesan cheese to taste
1 sprig of parsley or dill
Preheat the oven to 425ºF or 220ºC. Wash
potatoes well without peeling. Place potatoes
on a baking tray covered with tin foil. Prick
the potatoes on all sides with a fork and smear
them with a mixture of oil and salt. Cook in
the oven for 1 hour or until soft. Remove the
flesh and mash. Separately sauté the onion,
mushrooms and white sauce in butter add the
potato puree and mix well. Stuff the potato
peel with this mixture, sprinkle with Parmesan
cheese and return to oven so that it may melt.
Garnish with parsley or dill. Serve hot.

# Menu # 47

**Celery and apple salad**
**Mexican squash soup**
**Soy hash**

## Celery and apple salad
4   sliced red apples
2   sliced sticks of celery
2   tbs. of grill sesame seeds
    Salt to taste
    Vinaigrette sauce to taste (see sauces)

Soak apples in water with lime drops for 15 minutes to prevent oxidation. Drain and mix all ingredients in a bowl and sprinkle with dressing and sesame seeds.

## Mexican squash soup
½   kilo of sliced Mexican squash
½   sliced leek
2   tbs. of oats
4   tbs. of chopped onion
1   crushed and chopped clove of garlic
1   tbs. of chopped celery
3   tbs. of vegetable oil
    Sea salt to taste

Cook squash with leek. When half cooked, remove from heat and add oats. Allow to cool and then blend. Sauté garlic, onion and celery, add blended squash and simmer for 10 minutes.

## Soy hash
1½   cup of textured soy meat for hash
1 cup of grated carrot
½   cup of grated chayote
1 cup of thinly sliced cabbage
1 cup of grated Mexican squash
¼   cup of seedless raisins
¼   cup of almonds, soaked, peeled and chopped
½   cup of diced candied citron
½   cup of olives or to taste
¼   cup of chopped capers
2 chopped bell peppers
1 finely chopped onion
3 finely chopped cloves of garlic
3 finely chopped red tomatoes
½ cup of orange juice
½ tsp. of cumin powder
3 fried Piquín chilies (cayenne)
Aromatic herbs: bay leaf, thyme and marjoram
Salt, pepper and garlic powder
Vegetable oil as needed

Place aromatic herbs (and/or all you have at home) in water and boil for 10 minutes. Remove and cook the soy in the same water for 5 minutes or until well hydrated. Drain thoroughly and fry until brown. Separately sauté garlic, onion and tomato, season for 5 minutes and add remaining ingredients and soy. Let season for 10 minutes. Serve hot. You may garnish with strips of avocado.

# Menu # 48

**Mixed salad**
**Pea soup**
**Entomatadas**
**Mixed salad**

1   cup of Cos lettuce in pieces
½   cup of finely chopped celery
1   sliced or chopped cucumber,
2   grated carrots
1   grated beetroots
2   sliced radishes
25 grams of grated fresh coconut or walnut
    Olive oil
    Lime juice

Arrange vegetables in a dish. Sprinkle with olive oil and lime, or your favorite dressing, and garnish with coconut.

**Pea soup**

1   handful of English peas per person
2   red tomatoes
½   leek
3   cloves of garlic
2   finely chopped Serrano chilies
½   handful of coriander (cilantro), or to taste
1   cup of water per person

Cook peas, leek, and coriander in water on a low heat. Blend one half of peas with all ingredients, except the Serrano chili. Sauté the mixture in oil and then add the remaining peas and the rest of the water in which they were cooked. Cook for 5 minutes. Serve with Serrano chili to taste.

**Entomatadas**

15 tortillas or to taste
6   grill red tomatoes
3   cloves of garlic
¼   onion
1   thinly sliced onion
1 cup of yogurt or curdled milk
    Oil as needed for frying
    Sea salt to taste

Blend tomato, garlic, and onion; strain and sauté in 2 tbs of oil, and condiment with salt. Dip the tortillas in the o hot oil and then dip by one in the tomato sauce. Fold or roll them to make tacos (you may fill them with cheese). Serve entomatadas garnished with yogurt, cheese and onion slices (you may garnish also with slices of radish).

# Menu # 49

**Lentil sprout salad**
**Squash flower soup**
**Strips of Poblano peppers with cheese**

### Lentil bean sprout salad

1    cup of lentil sprouts (see bean sprouts)
1    cup of finely chopped cilantro
4    tbs. of chopped parsley
5    tbs. of finely chopped celery
½    finely chopped large onion
2    finely chopped red tomatoes
3    sliced avocados
     Olive oil
     Lime juice to taste
     Soy sauce to taste
     Salt to taste
Mix all the ingredients.

### Squash flower soup

¾    kilo of squash flower
4    dry-fried (grill) red tomatoes
½    small onion
2    cloves of garlic
½    leek
100  grams of crumbled Chihuahua cheese
1½   liters of water or vegetable broth
Tortillas cut into small strips and fried
Oil as needed
Sea salt to taste

Blend tomato, garlic, onion, and leek, then strain. Sauté the mixture in oil and add water. When it comes to the boil, add squash flower and salt; season on a low heat for 10 minutes. Serve with cheese and tortillas.

### Poblano Pepper Strips with cheese

6    Poblano peppers
1 ½  thinly sliced onion
150  grams of Oaxaca cheese or
vegetarian cheese
150  grams of Chihuahua cheese
1    natural yogurt or skimmed milk
Vegetable oil
Sea salt to taste

Grill Poblano peppers and cover with a damp cloth for 1 hour so that they sweat; peel and remove veins and cut them into strips. Sauté onion and strips of chili in the oil and add yogurt and cheese. Condiment with salt to taste.

# Menu # 50

**Green bean salad**
**Chard soup**
**Wheat croquettes**

**Green bean salad**
2   cups of green beans cooked *al dente*
1   cup of peeled and chopped tomato
½   cup of sliced red onion
1   chopped Jalapeño chili
1   chopped clove of garlic
**Dressing:**

1   lime (juice)
1   orange (juice)
¼   tsp. of cumin powder
¼   tsp of ground coriander seeds
¼   cup of olive oil
    Salt to taste
Cut string beans into small pieces and mix with remaining ingredients. Let season with dressing.

**Chard soup**
½   kilo of chard
½   cup of semolina
½   cup of finely chopped leek
4   tbs. of chopped onion
2   tsp. of chopped garlic
4   tbs. of vegetable oil
6   cups of water or as necessary
Sea salt to taste
Cook leek in 2 cups of water for 15 minutes. Add chard, already washed and blended raw with the rest of the water. Brown semolina, onion and garlic in oil and add blended chard and salt. Let season for 10 minutes on a low heat.

Note: chard may be substituted by other vegetable.

**Wheat croquettes**
3   cups of wheat
1   finely chopped bell pepper
4   tbs. of chopped onion
4   tbs. of grated carrot
2   tbs. of finely chopped celery
3   tbs. of finely chopped parsley
3   tbs. of chopped coriander (cilantro)
2   tbs. of soy sauce
2   tbs. of wheat germ
1   cup of cottage cheese
2   eggs or chickpea flour
    Vegetable oil as needed
    Sea salt to taste
Wash wheat and soak for 12 hours. Then cook in the same water until it bursts (use the water used for cooking the wheat for the soup). Grind the wheat while hot with the eggs and mix all the ingredients. Make croquettes and fry them in hot oil.
Note: may also be served with red tomato salad, etcetera.

# Menu # 51

**Potato and celery salad**
**Broccoli with avocado sauce**
**Potato tortilla without egg**

### Potato and celery salad
1    kilo of cooked and diced potatoes
¾    cup of finely chopped celery
4    tbs. of mayonnaise without egg or
to taste
1    tsp. of oregano
6    leaves of Romaine lettuce
2    thinly sliced red tomatoes
    Olives to taste
    Salt to taste
Mix the potatoes, celery, onion, oregano and mayonnaise. Serve on the lettuce leaves and garnish with tomato and olives.
You may add another dressing if you wish.

### Broccoli with avocado sauce
3    bunches of broccoli
2    ripe avocados
    Sea salt to taste
½    lime (juice)
Cut the broccoli into small pieces and steam for a few minutes until tender. Peel avocados and mash with a fork, mixing it with lime juice and a pinch of salt. Serve broccoli in a bowl and pour the avocado sauce on top.

### Potato tortilla without egg
3    medium-size sliced potatoes
1    medium-size sliced onion
½    sliced Mexican squash
    Chickpea flour (you may also use soy, rice or corn flour, but chickpea give the best results
    Vegetable oil as needed
    Sea salt to taste
Sauté the potatoes, onion, and squash in a pan with hot oil and add salt to taste. Mix flour with water (60% and 40%, approximately one glass or a bit more for one tortilla)) in a separate bowl; add a pinch of salt and black pepper to taste and beat the mixture thoroughly to prevent lumps forming. You may also add a small tomato and chopped fresh parsley to make it juicier. When the potatoes and vegetables are cooked, mash them well, add chickpea flour and stir well. Place the dough in a pan with hot oil and move the pan prevent the dough from sticking. Then turn over to cook the other side and it is ready. It is advisable to let the tortilla cool a while before serving so that it does not break up when it is hot.

# Menu # 52

**Spinach salad**
**Bean soup**
**Tzotobilchay**

### Spinach salad
- Leaves of tender spinach to taste
- Chopped onion to taste
- Avocado to taste
- Parsley to taste
- Salt to taste

Wash spinach well and chop. Mix all ingredients. Garnish with lime, olive oil and salt, or with your favorite dressing.

### Bean soup
2   cups of cooked black beans
2   grill red tomatoes
1   Serrano chili
1   small piece of onion
½   chopped onion
4   tbs. of chopped coriander (cilantro)
1   cup of cottage cheese o curd cheese
4   tbs. of vegetable oil
    Sea salt to taste
5   tortillas cut into strips and fried (chips)

Blend the tomatoes, onion and Serrano chili; strain and sauté in oil. Blend beans, strain and add to the sauce with the broth in which they were cooked. Let season at a low heat for 15 minutes. Add cheese, chopped onion, coriander, and tortilla chips to serve.

### Tzotobilchay
1    kilo of corn dough
½    kilo of chopped chaya or chard,
½    liter of vegetable oil
     Sea salt to taste
6    chopped hard-boiled eggs
200  grams of ground pumpkin seeds
1    onion
4    grill red tomatoes
1    Piquín chili or to taste
     Banana leaves

To prepare the sauce, blend the tomato, onion and chili, strain and sauté in 2 spoonfuls of oil and condiment with salt.

Mix the dough, oil, salt and previously washed chaya or chard separately. Knead well. Spread a piece of the dough over pieces of the banana leaves, sprinkle ground pumpkin seeds, a small amount of egg and sauce. Wrap the dough tightly in the banana leaves and press well and then steam. You may also make the dough into a single roll that you can slice when serving. You can sprinkle ground seeds and sauce on each slice (as you can with the smaller portions).

**Note:** if you use corn flour, blend a piece of onion in a little hot salted water and add to flour; it will improve the flavor of the dough. To sear banana leaves, pass them quickly over the heat on one side only and cut to the desired size.

# Menu # 53

**Eggplant salad**
**Gazpacho**
**Poblano peppers stuffed with soy meat**

## Eggplant salad

2    eggplants
½    finely chopped onion,
2    peeled and chopped red tomatoes
1    finely chopped green pepper
3    sliced hard-boiled eggs (optional)
4    tbs. of soy sauce
2    tbs. of olive oil
     Salt and pepper to taste

Cut eggplants into four pieces, cook in a little water and oil and then peel and mash. Mix the eggplants with the other ingredients and garnish with sliced egg or red pepper.
Note: may also be served as side dish.

## Gazpacho

1    kilo of red tomatoes
2    diced cucumbers
2    diced avocados
2    tbs. of Tabasco sauce
1    pinch of brown sugar
     Olive oil to taste
     Salt and pepper to taste
     Apple vinegar to taste

Blend tomatoes raw and strain. Condiment with salt, and pepper to taste and add remaining ingredients. Serve very cold, together with whole wheat Havana cookies.

## Poblano peppers stuffed with soy meat

8    washed and grilled poblano peppers
2    cups of textured soy, already prepared or finely chopped wheat gluten
1    cup of mayonnaise
3    tsp. of mustard
1    large sliced onion
4    chopped cloves of garlic
¼    cup of olive oil
3    tbs. of lime juice
     Aromatic herbs: bay leaf, marjoram and thyme
Sea salt to taste

Sauté soy meat in a little oil until brown. Add mayonnaise and mustard and stuff the peppers with this mixture. Sauté the garlic and onion in ¼ cup of olive oil; add lime, salt and aromatic herbs and season for 5 minutes. Remove from the heat and cover saucepan. Stand for 15 minutes. Place peppers in a dish and sprinkle with this blend. Refrigerate until served.

# Menu # 54

**Arabian salad**
**Mushroom soup**
**Baked chayotes**

**Arabian salad**

| | |
|---|---|
| 1 | finely chopped red tomato |
| ½ | finely chopped onion |
| 1 | finely chopped clove of garlic |
| 3 | finely chopped sprigs of parsley |
| 2 | finely chopped sprigs of mint |
| 1 | finely chopped cucumber |
| 1 | finely chopped green chilies |
| 2 | limes (juice) |
| 4 | tbs. of olive oil |
| | Salt to taste |

Mix all ingredients. The mixture should be slightly runny. You may add ½ cup of cooked chickpeas.

**Mushroom soup**

| | |
|---|---|
| 1 | kilo of mushrooms (varied) washed and chopped |
| ½ | finely chopped onion |
| 1 | sprig of epazote |
| 6 | cups of water or as needed |
| 1 | clove of garlic or to taste |
| | Salt and pepper to taste |

Sauté garlic and onion, add mushrooms and sauté for just a moment. Add water, salt and pepper. Add epazote when the saucepan comes to the boil. You may give it a spicy touch by adding chipotle chili.

Note: tastes better when reheated the day after.

**Baked chayotes**

| | |
|---|---|
| 4 | medium-size chayotes |
| 2 | chopped red tomatoes |
| 1 | chopped small onion |
| 2 | chopped cloves of garlic |
| 2 | cups of kernel corn |
| 3 | tbs. of yogurt or curdled milk |
| 3 | tbs. of butter or vegetarian margarine |
| 200 | grams of Chihuahua cheese or |
| | Vegetarian cheese |
| | Sea salt to taste |

Cook chayotes whole and with the peel. Allow to cool and then cut in half long ways, scoop out part of the flesh with a spoon, mash and add the curdled milk. Cook the corn on its own. Sauté garlic, onion, tomato, and corn. Mix with the flesh of the chayotes and stuff the chayote halves; place cheese and butter on top. Place in a dish and bake until melted.

# Menu # 55

**Beetroot salad**
**Green rice**
**Stuffed Mexican squash**

**Beetroot salad**

2    cups of grated or cooked
     and diced raw beetroot,
2    tsp of finely chopped onion
¼    of natural yogurt or sour cream
1    tbs. of lime juice
1    tbs. of olive oil
     Grated fresh coconut
     Sea salt to taste

Mix all ingredients and garnish with fresh coconut.

**Green rice**

1    cup or whole grain rice
3    cups of water
2    grilled and washed poblano peppers
2    cups of kernel corn
2    sprigs of epazote
3    sprigs of coriander (cilantro)
3    sprigs of parsley
¼    onion
2    cloves of garlic
4    tbs. of vegetable oil
     Sea salt to taste

Wash rice well. Boil in water for three minutes; rinse in cold water and drain. Fry the rice with the corn until light brown. Blend chilies, garlic, onion, coriander and parsley with a little water and add to the rice with epazote and the rest of the water; condiment with salt. When it comes to the boil, cover and simmer fire for around 45 minutes.

**Stuffed Mexican squash**

7    round squash
5    grated carrots or huitlacoche
¼    cup of finely chopped coriander
½    finely chopped onion
½    cup of chopped walnuts
½    cup of soy milk
½    cup of Fresh or Chihuahua cheese
1    natural yogurt
1    tbs. of chopped garlic
1    tbs. of whole grain flour
4    tbs. of oil
     Salt to taste

Cook squash in a little water, cut off the top part and remove the inner part with a teaspoon. Sauté: garlic, onion, carrots, coriander, and flesh of the squash. Add salt to taste. Remove from the heat and add cheese. Stuff the squash. If you wish, bake for 5 minutes.

# Menu # 56

**Cesar salad**
**Vegetarian lasagna**
**Soy meat with xoconoxtle**

### Cesar salad
1   Wash Cos or Romaine lettuce
½   sliced shallot or red onion
2   crushed and chopped cloves of garlic
1   tbs. of strong mustard
1   tbs. of chopped fresh parsley
3   tbs. of apple vinegar
½   cup of olive oil
1   egg yolk
¼   cup of Parmesan cheese
    Several drops of lime juice
    Salt and pepper to taste
    Homemade garlic croutons

Mix the garlic, onion, mustard, parsley, vinegar and yolk and stir well. Add oil in a steady flow while whipping with blender; add several drops of lime. The sauce should be thick. Cut lettuce by hand into large pieces and place in a bowl. Pour vinaigrette on top and mix well. Add croutons and sprinkle with cheese. Serve immediately.

### Vegetarian lasagna
½   kilo of lasagna pasta
3   tbs. of vegetable oil or as needed
2   diced carrots
1   diced Mexican squash
½   finely chopped cauliflower
1   finely chopped green pepper
1   finely chopped onion
2   peeled and chopped red tomatoes
1   cup of chopped champignons
½   tbs. of grated lime peel
¼   tsp. of nutmeg

½   tsp. of grounded clove
½   tsp. of oregano
¼   tsp of thyme
1   cup of grated Gruyere cheese
1   cup of grated Mozzarella cheese
4   cups of light white sauce (see sauces)
    Sea salt and pepper to taste

Preheat oven to at 190ºC or 375ºF. Cook pasta *al dente* in a wide saucepan with salted water and a little oil. Drain and place the strips of lasagna.

Sauté the onion, add the carrots and cook for 3 minutes. Add remaining vegetables and finally the tomatoes, mushrooms and spices. Simmer for 4 minutes. Remove from heat, cover and stand. Place a layer of pasta in a greased dish, followed by a layer of vegetables, a layer of cheese and white sauce. Repeat layers until you end up with a layer of pasta on top. Add sauce and cover with cheese. Bake for 30 minutes.

### Soy meat with xoconoxtle
¼   kilo of vegetable soy meat
2   xoconoxtles
1   small onion
2   cloves of garlic
4   tbs. of vegetable oil
1   Serrano chili
1   cup of vegetable broth
    Aromatic herbs
    Oil as needed
    Sea salt to taste

Cook previously soaked soy meat with ¾ of onion and aromatic herbs. Drain well and fry until brown. Peel the xoconox.tle and remove the seeds from the middle. Blend the garlic, onion, xoconoxtle and chili with the broth. Sauté this sauce in oil and add the meat. Let season with salt and simmer for 15 minutes. Remove from heat and allow standing.

# Menu # 57

**Italian salad**
**Pozole with mushrooms**
**Corn cupcakes**

### Italian salad
1    chopped Cos lettuce,
1    chopped bunch of spinach
2    finely chopped sticks of celery,
3    chopped red tomatoes
1    chopped small red onion
2    diced avocados
Mix all the ingredients and pour the dressing on top.

### Dressing:
1    lime (juice)
1    orange (juice)
1    grapefruit (juice)
4    tbs. of olive oil or to taste
     Oregano to taste
     Sea salt to taste

### Corn cupcakes
1¼   cup of whole wheat flour
¾    cup of corn flour
1    cup of soy milk
½    cup of raisins
⅓    cup of oil
3    tsp. of baking powder
½    tsp. of salt
4    Tbs. of bee's honey or to taste
3    eggs
Preheat the oven to 200ºC. Sift the dry ingredients and blend liquid ingredients and then mix the two. Add raisins coated with flour. Use a spoon to place the pieces of dough in small molds already greased and covered with flour. Bake cupcakes for 15 minutes.

### Pozole with mushrooms
½    kilo of cooked hominy
¾    kilo of sliced mushrooms
2    Guajillo chilies with the veins removed
     and boiled with onion
1    Pasilla chili (as above)
3    grill red tomatoes
3    cloves of garlic
½    small onion
Sea salt to taste
To prepare the sauce: blend the chilies, tomatoes, onion, and garlic with the corn broth. Sieve and sauté in oil, add the oregano, salt, and simmer for 10 minutes. Pour this sauce on the hominy in the water in which it was cooked and season 10 minutes. Add mushrooms and boil for 5 minutes.
Serve with a garnish of:
*   Finely chopped onion,
*   Thinly sliced radish
*   Chopped lettuce
*   Oregano
*   Lime to taste

# Menu # 58

**Mixed salad**
**Lentil bean sprout soup**
**Eggplant soufflé**

## Mixed salad
½   washed lettuce and cut into pieces
2-3  sliced red tomatoes
1   sliced cucumber
2   grated carrots
Lime or apple vinegar
Olive oil and salt to taste
Or your favorite dressing
Place all vegetables in a dish and pour the dressing on top.

## Lentil bean sprout soup
2   cups of lentil bean sprouts (see bean sprouts)
3   grilled red tomatoes
½   chopped leek
¼   medium-size onion
2   cloves of garlic
6   cups of water, or as needed
    Aromatic herbs
Blend the tomatoes, onion and garlic; strain and sauté. Add lentils, leek, water and aromatic herbs. Simmer for 15 minutes or until lentils are cooked.
Note: add vegetables to taste.

## Eggplant soufflé
4    medium-size eggplants
1    cup of cooked whole grain rice
4    tomatoes
½    onion
3    cloves of garlic
1    chopped bell pepper
5    tbs. of chopped parsley
200  grams of grated Chihuahua cheese
100  grams of grated panela cheese
2    plain yogurts
Cut eggplants into slices and leave for one hour in cold salted water. Blend the tomatoes, onion and garlic and strain and sauté in a little oil. Add salt, pepper and parsley and simmer for 4 minutes. Place layers of the eggplant, rice, tomato sauce and cheese in a greased dish and top with eggplant, sauce, cheese and yogurt. Bake until melted for about 20 minutes.

# Menu # 59

**Spinach salad**
**Carrot cream (Soup)**
**Huitlacoche crepes**

**Spinach salad**

3 cups of chopped spinach or to taste
1½ cups of sliced palmettos
1 cup of sliced mushrooms
½ cup of red onion or shallot (a hybrid of onion and garlic)
¼ kilo of cherry-red tomato
4 loaves of bread, diced
Wash vegetables well. Place in a salad bowl and season with vinaigrette dressing or your favorite dressing (see dressings). Garnish with croutons (toasted bread fried in olive oil).

**Carrot cream soup**

7 sliced carrots
1 cup of sliced leek
1 small potato
½ cup of celery
½ cup of finely chopped parsley
6 cups of water or as needed
2 hard-boiled eggs (optional)
4 tbs. of olive oil
Sea salt and pepper to taste
Cook the carrots, leek and potato; blend with the water used for cooking and 2 egg yolks. Sauté in oil and add remaining broth; the mixture should be slightly thick. Condiment with salt and simmer for 5 minutes. Add celery and cook for 1 minute more. Serve with chopped egg whites and parsley.

**Huitlacoche crepes**
**Crepes (see crepes)**
**Filling:**

1 kg. of huitlacoche cut in small pieces
1 cup of kernel corn, cooked
1 finely chopped onion
3 crushed and chopped cloves of garlic,
3 chopped sprigs of epazote,
2 Serrano chilies or o to taste
25 grams of manchego or Chihuahua or vegetarian cheese
1 cup of cream or natural yogurt
Sea salt to taste
Sauté garlic and onion and then add chilies, huitlacoche, corn, epazote and salt. Cover and simmer until the juice has dried.

**Sauce:**

9 grilled and washed poblano peppers
¼ onion
1 clove of garlic
¾ cup of cow or soy milk
4 tbs. of vegetable oil
Blend ingredients and sauté in oil, season. Stuff crepes with huitlacoche and roll. Place in greased dish. Bathe with sauce, cream and grated cheese. Bake until melted.

# Menu # 60

**Mixed salad**
**Cream of onion soup**
**Vegetarian codfish**

### Mixed salad
1   Romaine lettuce
2   sliced red tomatoes,
2   thinly sliced sticks of celery
2   sliced avocados
Break the lettuce into pieces and wash. Place vegetables in a bowl and add dressing as desired (see dressings).

### Cream of onion soup
2   sliced onions
5   cups of vegetable broth or to taste
¼   kg. of grated Chihuahua or Oaxaca cheese
5   tbs. of olive oil
Sauté the onion in oil until transparent, then blend ⅔ of the onion in the broth. Pour on the remaining onion, season with salt and boil; add more broth if necessary. Serve hot over cheese, which must be at the bottom of the dish.

### Vegetarian codfish
½   kilo of vegetable meat already prepared (textured soy)
10  crushed cloves of garlic
3   chopped onions
2   kgs. of peeled, chopped red tomato
1   bunch of finely chopped parsley
1   can of bell pepper (red)
1   can of large chilies
1   flask of olives
1   flask of capers
1   fried French bread
Sea weeds to taste
½   cup of olive oil or to taste
    Sea Salt to taste
Fry garlic in oil until brown and then remove. Sauté the onion and tomato in the same oil season well and add prepared textured soy and cut into little pieces. Blend the garlic, pepper and bread and then add to the soy. Simmer for 30 minutes; stir constantly to avoid the mixture sticking. Add olives, capers and parsley. Add sea weed. Stand and serve with large chilies. It is delicious.

# Sauces And Dressings And More...

## Elianne vinaigrette

| Ingredients | Preparation |
|---|---|
| ¾ cup of virgin olive oil<br>⅛ cup of apple vinegar<br>⅛ cup of soy sauce<br>3 crushed and chopped cloves of garlic<br>To taste: sliced onion, finely chopped parsley, Worcestershire sauce. (optional) | Mix all ingredients and marinate. This is delicious vinaigrette. You may refrigerate for several weeks. You may add finely chopped olives. |

## Vinaigrette (basic recipe)

| Ingredients | Preparation |
|---|---|
| 1 small clove garlic, peeled<br>½ cup cider vinegar or fresh lemon juice<br>1 shallot, minced<br>1 tsp Dijon mustard (optional)<br>1 cup extra virgin olive oil<br>3 pinches of sea salt or to taste<br>Ground black pepper to taste | Shake well.<br>Taste and adjust the seasonings. Use at once or cover and refrigerate. |

## Fresh herb vinaigrette

| Preparation |
|---|
| Prepare basic vinaigrette. Adding 1/3 cup minced or finely snipped fresh herbs: basil, parsley, dill, thyme and chives. |

## Honey mustard vinaigrette

| Ingredients | Preparation |
|---|---|
| 2 Tbsp fresh lemon juice<br>1 Tbsp cider vinegar<br>1 tsp honey or to taste<br>1 tsp whole grain mustard or to taste<br>6 Tbsp extra virgin olive oil<br>Sea salt an black pepper to taste | Shake well.<br>Taste and adjust the seasoning.<br>Use immediately or cover and refrigerate. |

## Vinaigrette

| Ingredients | Preparation |
|---|---|
| ¾ cup of virgin olive oil<br>⅛ cup of apple vinegar or lime juice<br>1 finely chopped clove of garlic<br>½ tbs. of mustard<br>2 tbs. of chopped parsley<br>1 tbs. of chopped mint<br>½ tsp. of thyme<br>1 tsp. of brown sugar<br>Salt and pepper to taste | Mix all ingredients in a glass jar; cover it and shake well until well blended. Ready to serve. |

## Spanish vinaigrette

| Ingredients | Preparation |
|---|---|
| 2 tbs. of apple vinegar<br>6 tbs. of olive oil<br>3 tbs. of soy sauce<br>1 tbs. of chopped capers<br>1 tbs. of chopped parsley<br>½ tsp. of grounded thyme<br>½ tsp. of grounded marjoram<br>1 bay leaf<br>½ finely chopped bell pepper<br>1 finely chopped hard-boiled egg<br>Salt and pepper to taste | Mix all ingredients. |

## Marinade vegetables

| Ingredients | Preparation |
|---|---|
| 1 ½ cups vegetable oil<br>1 ½ cups cider vinegar<br>2 Tbsp red wine (optional)<br>2 red onions, sliced<br>2 cloves garlic, crushed<br>1 tsp soy sauce<br>Garden herbs, such as basil and oregano<br>Sea salt and pepper to taste | Mix well all the ingredients. |

## Asian style marinade

| Ingredients | Preparation |
|---|---|
| ½ cup cider vinegar<br>1 Tbsp light sesame oil<br>¼ cup honey<br>1 clove garlic, crushed<br>2 inch piece ginger root, peeled and grated<br>1/4 cup pineapple juice | Mix well all the ingredients.<br>Use this marinade is great for:<br>Asparagus, broccoli, carrots, beets, onions, mushrooms and tofu |

## Citrus herb marinade

| Ingredients | Preparation |
|---|---|
| ¼ cup olive oil and sesame oil<br>2 ½ Tbsp fresh lemon juice<br>1 ½ Tbsp fresh orange juice<br>1 ½ tsp dried thyme leaves<br>1/3 cup fresh parsley, finely chopped<br>½ bay leaf, very finely crumbled<br>1 clove garlic, minced<br>Sea salt to taste<br>Ground white pepper to taste | Combine in a bowl and blend with a fork.<br>Use immediately, or cover and refrigerate for up to one week. |

## Mediterranean garlic marinade

| Ingredients | Preparation |
|---|---|
| ½ cup olive oil<br>¼ cup cider or balsamic vinegar<br>¼ cup red onion, minced<br>1 clove garlic, crushed<br>2 cups mixed fresh herbs: parsley, sage, rosemary, thyme, basil and oregano<br>Sea salt and ground black pepper to taste | Mix all the ingredients.<br>This sauce is recommended for marinate:<br>Asparagus, artichoke hearts, broccoli, tomatoes, eggplant, onions, leeks, mushrooms, zucchini and tofu |

## Yogurt marinade

| Ingredients | Preparation |
|---|---|
| 1 cup nonfat plain yogurt<br>2 cloves garlic, peeled and grated<br>2 Tbsp lemon juice<br>2 inch piece ginger root, peeled and grated<br>¼ cup cilantro, minced<br>1 Tbsp curry powder<br>2 tsp ground cumin | Mix well all the ingredients.<br>Use this marinade for:<br>Eggplant, potatoes, tomatoes, mushrooms and tofu. |

## Moroccan spice oil

| Ingredients | Spice grinder (an inexpensive coffee |
|---|---|
| ½ cup extra virgin olive oil | Grinder will do) or mortar and pestle |
| 2 tsp whole cumin seeds | and grind with cinnamon, ginger and red |
| 2 tsp whole coriander seeds | pepper flakes. |
| 1 tsp whole fennel seeds | Return spices to a pot; add oil and heat |
| 1 tsp ground cinnamon | just until oil is warmed through 1 or 2 |
| 1 tsp ground ginger | minutes. Strain oil through a fine meshed |
| ½ tsp red pepper flakes | strainer lined with cheesecloth and store in |
| Preparation | tightly closer jar. |
| Toast cumin, coriander an fennel seeds, | Mix well all the ingredients. |
| about 3 minutes (be careful not to burn | Just a drizzle of this spicy oil added to |
| spices). Immediately transfer seeds to | beans, grains or vegetables will turn them |
| | into exciting fare. |

## Light white sauce

| Ingredients | Preparation |
|---|---|
| 2 cups of hot milk | Add the flour to the butter and cook for |
| 2 tbs. of butter | 2 minutes. Add milk gradually and stir to |
| 2 tbs. of flour | prevent lumps forming; add salt, pepper and |
| Salt and white pepper to taste | season at a low heat for 10 minutes, stirring |
| Grated Cheddar or Mozzarella cheese and | constantly. |
| nutmeg to taste | |

## White oat sauce

| Ingredients | Preparation |
|---|---|
| ½ cup of oats | Blend oats dry. Sauté onion in hot butter and |
| 2 tbs. of butter | then add oats. Add milk gradually, stirring |
| ½ finely chopped onion | constantly. Season and cook for 2 minutes at |
| 1 cup of milk (cow or soy) | a low heat. |
| 1 pinch of nutmeg | |
| Salt to taste | |

## Béchamel sauce (basic white sauce)

| Ingredients | Preparation |
|---|---|
| 10 tbs. of melted butter | Dissolve the flour and butter in a cup of milk |
| 10 tbs. of flour | and cook at a low heat. Pour in the rest of |
| 5 cups of milk | the milk and stir constantly. Condiment with |
| Salt and nutmeg | salt and nutmeg and boil for 3 minutes. |
| Variant: instead of butter use olive oil, and | Variant: when the béchamel sauce is hot, |
| instead of cow's milk use soy milk. Add a | add ½ cup of Parmesan cheese and cook for |
| finely chopped onion and sauté. | another 2 minutes. Add mushrooms if you |
| | wish. |

## Tartar sauce

| Ingredients | Preparation |
|---|---|
| 1 tbs. of mustard<br>3 finely chopped pickles<br>1 tsp. of chopped chives<br>1 tbs. of finely chopped parsley<br>2 tbs. of chopped capers<br>2 tsp. of juice of lime<br>4 finely chopped hard-boiled eggs<br>Tabasco sauce to taste<br>Salt and pepper to taste | Mix all ingredients and refrigerate until served. |

## Pasta sauce

| Ingredients | Preparation |
|---|---|
| 4 peeled and chopped red tomatoes<br>2 cups of tomato paste<br>2 finely chopped cloves of garlic<br>½ cup of finely chopped onions<br>1 cup of sliced mushrooms<br>½ cup of finely chopped olives<br>½ cup of finely chopped celery<br>½ cup of finely chopped parsley<br>¼ cup of chopped carrot (optional)<br>¼ tsp. of oregano<br>¼ tsp. of tarragon<br>1 tsp. of salt<br>2 tbs. of brown sugar<br>2 tbs. of whole wheat flour<br>1 pinch of sweet pepper<br>1 pinch of cinnamon<br>¼ of cup of oil<br>Aromatic herbs<br>Worcestershire sauce to taste | Sauté onion, garlic, carrot and celery. Allow to simmer and sprinkle flour and add tomato, mushrooms and spices. Simmer for 30 minutes. Add parsley and olives. Serve with spaghetti or any kind of cooked and hot pasta; sprinkle Parmesan cheese on top.<br>Note: another type of pasta sauce is made from milk cream, butter, saffron, Parmesan, pepper and salt. |

## Tomato ketchup

| Ingredients | Preparation |
|---|---|
| 1     liter of tomato paste<br>¼   kg. finely chopped onion<br>1     tbs. of mustard<br>1     tbs. of salt<br>1     tbs. of pepper<br>½   tsp. of grounded clove<br>1     pinch of cayenne pepper<br>1     cinnamon stick<br>½   cup of apple vinegar<br>4     crushed cloves of garlic<br>2     bay leaves<br>100 grams of brown sugar<br>1     pinch of red vegetable coloring (optional) | Mix all ingredients and cook at a very low heat for ½ hour, stirring occasionally. Keep in sterilized flasks and seal with cork and wax.<br>For paste: wash tomatoes and cut into pieces, cook until tender; strain through a strainer and then through a cloth. |

## Tomato sauce (basic recipe)

| Ingredients | Preparation |
|---|---|
| 4 cups fresh tomatoes, peeled and coarsely chopped<br>1 Tbsp tomato paste (optional)<br>½ cup fresh parsley, finely chopped<br>3 cloves garlic, minced<br>1 medium red onion, finely chopped<br>1 celery stalk with leaves, chopped<br>½ cup fresh basil leaves, chopped<br>1 tsp spring herb each: fresh rosemary, oregano, sage and thyme<br>4 Tbsp extra virgin olive oil<br>1 carrot, peeled and finely chopped<br>Sea salt and pepper to taste | Combine together all the ingredients. Cook over very low heat, stirring frequently for about 10-15 minutes, until the sauce is thickened.<br>Remove the herb springs. |

## Mexican sauce

| Ingredients | Preparation |
|---|---|
| ¼ cup Serrano chilies, diced<br>8 diced leeks<br>1 cup fresh cilantro, finely chopped<br>5 medium-size tomatoes, chopped<br>2 cloves garlic, minced<br>1 cup fresh tomato, peeled, seeded, juicy and chopped<br>½ large white or red onion, chopped<br>Juice of ½ lime. | Mix all the ingredients and refrigerate 2-3 hours to develop flavor. |

## Lentil sauce

| Ingredients | Preparation |
|---|---|
| ¾ cup of lentil bean sprouts<br>¼ cup of onion cut in four pieces<br>¼ cup of tomato sauce<br>1 crushed and chopped clove of garlic<br>2 tbs. of lime juice<br>5 tbs. of green tomato sauce<br>1 tsp. of grounded cumin<br>1½ tsp. of piquin chili<br>½ tsp. of sea salt | Cook lentils, garlic and onion and then strain. Keep the broth for soups. Blend all ingredients. Refrigerate until thick. It is very tasty.<br>Note: serve on raw or steamed vegetables. |

## Corn sauce

| Ingredients | Preparation |
|---|---|
| 2 cups of cooked tender kernel corn<br>1 cup of finely chopped red onion<br>3 finely chopped cloves of garlic,<br>2 red or yellow peppers, dry-fried, washed and finely chopped<br>1 finely chopped Jalapeño peppers<br>2 limes (juice)<br>¼ cup of olive oil or to taste<br>½ tsp. of grounded cumin<br>Chopped cilantro to taste<br>Salt and pepper to taste. | Mix all ingredients. Serve on top of gluten meat steaks, roast potatoes, etcetera. |

## Chimichurri sauce (basic recipe)

| Ingredients | Preparation |
|---|---|
| ½ cup olive oil<br>¼ cup apple vinegar<br>1 small red onion, finely chopped<br>1/3 cup fresh parsley, cilantro and finely chopped<br>4 cloves garlic, finely chopped<br>Sea salt to taste<br>Ground red pepper to taste<br>Ground black pepper to taste | Mix well all the ingredients.<br>Cover and let stand for 3 hours before serving to allow the flavors to develop. This sauce will keep, covered and refrigerate for up to 2-4 days. |

## Chimichurri sauce

| Ingredients | Preparation |
|---|---|
| For one liter:<br>10   sprigs of finely chopped parsley<br>5   finely chopped garlic bulbs<br>1   liter of sunflower oil<br>½   liter of olive oil<br>5   seedless dry-ground guajillo chilies<br>1   cup of apple vinegar<br>2   tbs. of salt<br>1½ cups of boiling water | Mix parsley, garlic, and chili with the oils and vinegar. Add boiling water and salt. Allow to stand. |

## Italian pesto

| Ingredients | Preparation |
|---|---|
| 4 plum tomatoes, peeled, seeded and chopped<br>2 cloves garlic, chopped<br>½ cup blanched almonds, roughly chopped<br>½ cup basil leaves<br>1 Tbsp extra virgin olive oil<br>Sea salt and pepper to taste | Place tomatoes, garlic almonds and basil in blender or food processor or mortar.<br>Drizzle in oil; process or grind with pestle until pureed to desired consistency (almonds should still provide a little crunch). Add salt and pepper to taste.<br>Serve over cooked pasta if desired.<br>Make about one cup. |

## Pine nut pesto (basic recipe)

| Ingredients | Preparation |
|---|---|
| 2 cups fresh basil leaves<br>½ cup olive oil<br>1/3 cup pine nuts, toasted<br>2-3 cloves garlic peeled<br>½ tsp sea salt | Place basil and olive oil in a food processor or blender and blend until smooth.<br>Add remaining ingredients and blend until smooth. Do not over blend or it will get hot and separate. |

## Pesto sauce

| Ingredients | Preparation |
|---|---|
| 2 cups fresh basil leaves<br>½ cup pine nuts<br>3 medium cloves garlic, peeled<br>½ cup grated Parmesan cheese or soy Parmesan cheese<br>¾ cup extra virgin olive oil<br>Sea salt and pepper to taste | Place in fool processor or blender and blend all the ingredients.<br>Use immediately or store in a covered glass jar in refrigerator. |

## Pesto

| Ingredients | Preparation |
|---|---|
| 2 handfuls of chopped basil with leaves and flower<br>150 grams of chopped pecans or pine nuts<br>2 crushed and chopped cloves of garlic<br>Olive oil to taste<br>Grape seeds oil to taste<br>Salt to taste | Wash basil well. Mix all ingredients. Cover with oil to preserve.<br><br>Note: you may use parsley instead of basil. All the ingredients are usually blended. |

## Low-fat pesto

| c | Preparation |
|---|---|
| **1 cup fresh basil leaves, chopped**<br>**¾ cup fresh parsley, chopped**<br>**1 Tbsp grated style soy cheese**<br>**1-2 cloves garlic, minced**<br>**2 Tbsp white miso**<br>**Water the necessary**<br>**1/3 cup toasted bread** | **Place all the ingredients, except water in a food processor or blender, and blend until minced; add water to desired consistency.** |

## Sesame seed sauce

| Ingredients | Preparation |
|---|---|
| ¾ cup of toasted sesame seeds<br>2 finely chopped red tomatoes<br>3 cloves of garlic<br>½ cup of chopped parsley or to taste<br>½ cup of water<br>1 lime (juice)<br>Sea salt to taste | Blend sesame seeds, garlic, lime juice, salt and water. Mix with remaining ingredients and serve. |

## Alioli

| Ingredients | Preparation |
|---|---|
| 5 crushed cloves of garlic<br>2 egg yolks<br>1 cup of olive oil<br>½ tsp. of lime juice<br>Tabasco sauce to taste<br>Sea salt to taste | Crush garlic with the sauce in a stone mortar. Blend all ingredients until thick. |

## Roquefort dressing

| Ingredients | Preparation |
| --- | --- |
| 1     cup of plain yogurt<br>7     almonds<br>2     cloves of garlic<br>      Roquefort cheese to taste<br>      Soy sauce to taste | Blend all ingredients. Serve on watercress salad, or your favorite one. |

## Pecan sauce (Nogada)

| Ingredients | Preparation |
| --- | --- |
| 2     cups of pecans (halves)<br>1     cup of washed almonds<br>1     cream cheese<br>      Sour cream or yogurt to taste | Blend all ingredients. Delicious. |

## Citric dressing

| Ingredients | Preparation |
| --- | --- |
| To taste:<br>Orange juice<br>Grapefruit juice<br>Lime juice<br>Grounded aniseed, garlic powder and salt | Mix all ingredients. |

## Tofu dressing

| Ingredients | Preparation |
| --- | --- |
| 250   grams of diced tofu<br>200   grams of cottage cheese<br>1¼    cup of plain yogurt or sour cream<br>1      tbs. of pumpkin seeds<br>1      lime (juice)<br>1      finely chopped small onion<br>1      pinch of brown sugar<br>1      tbs. of olive oil<br>Sea salt and pepper to taste<br>4      tbs. of finely chopped assorted herbs:<br>       basil, fresh cilantro, watercress and dill | Blend all ingredients except the herbs. Mix all ingredients. Serve with black bread.<br>Note: vary the herbs. |

## Humus be tjine

| Ingredients | Preparation |
|---|---|
| 2 cup chickpeas, cooked | Blend all ingredients (except olive oil) in a |
| ¼ cup lime juice or to taste | blender and blend until smooth and creamy. |
| ¼ cup sesame seed sauce (tahini) | Transfer hummus to serving plate and drizzle |
| 3-4 cloves garlic | with olive oil and curry powder (a little)' |
| ½ tsp sea salt | Serve with pitas (Arabian bread) |
| ¼ cup olive oil | Serve immediately or transfer to a storage |
| ¼ cup chickpea broth or necessary | container with lid and refrigerate until use. |
| ¼ tsp cumin | |
| ¼ tsp cider vinegar | |
| 15 pecans or to taste | |

## Tahini dressing

| Ingredients | Preparation |
|---|---|
| 1 cup tahini (sesame butter) | Mix all the ingredients in a bowl. Add sea |
| ½ cup water | salt and ground red pepper to taste. |
| Juice of 2 lemons, or to taste | Thin with water as necessary, especially when |
| 3 cloves garlic, minced | using as dressing. |
| 1 Tbsp fresh cilantro, minced or to taste | Taste and adjust the seasonings. |
| 1 tsp ground coriander | Use or refrigerate. |
| ½ tsp ground cumin | |

## Tjina

| Ingredients | Preparation |
|---|---|
| 5 tbs. of sesame paste (tahini) | Blend all the ingredients. |
| 5 tbs. of cold water | |
| 3 tbs. of lime juice | |
| Parsley and salt to taste | |

## Brown gravy

| Ingredients | Preparation |
|---|---|
| **1 Tbsp corn starch** | **Mix corn starch, soy sauce and vegetable** |
| **2 Tbsp soy sauce** | **seasoning together in sauce pan.** |
| **½ tsp vegetable seasoning** | **Gradually add water, stir well.** |
| **2 cups water** | **Cook over moderate heat until thick.** |
| **¼ tahini (sesame butter)** | **Add tahini. Mix well** |

## Gomasio

| Ingredients | Preparation |
|---|---|
| 7 to 12 tbs. of sesame seeds | Wash sesame seeds and toast lightly. |
| 3 to 6 tbs. of sea salt | Toast salt lightly separately. Allow to cool |
| | blend both ingredients dry. Place in a flask. |
| | Serve with salads, soups, stews, etcetera. |

## Ghee (clarified butter)

| Preparation |
|---|
| Boil salt-free butter for 10 minutes at a moderate heat. Remove from heat and stand for a few minutes before removing the white foam. The remaining transparent yellow liquid is the ghee. Pour in a container without draining the white sediment. Use instead of butter or oil. |

## Salt-free diet

| Ingredients | Preparation |
|---|---|
| 30 grams of sesame seeds<br>30 grams of millet seeds<br>10 grams of sea salt | Mix dry and place keep in a salt shaker. If there is insufficient salt, add toasted and grounded sesame seeds. |

## Broad bean or chickpeas falafel

| Ingredients | Preparation |
|---|---|
| 2 cups of dry broad beans or chickpeas soaked for 24 hours<br>To taste: cilantro, parsley, mint, Serrano chilies, lots of garlic and cumin. Breadcrumbs, salt and white pepper. | Blend all ingredients well with a little water to a thick consistency. Shape into small balls and fry in oil until brown. To serve, cut pita bread in half, open each one and stuff with falafel, tjina and vegetables to taste. |

## Paste for coating (special recipe)

| Ingredients | Preparation |
|---|---|
| ½ cup of white flour<br>¼ cup of whole meal flour<br>½ cup of wheat germ<br>1 egg<br>1 tsp. of baking powder<br>Warm water as needed | Place the flours and baking powder in a container; slowly add warm water and beat the mixture. Add egg and continue beating until achieving a fairly thick mixture. **Note:** you may use this paste to coat vegetables, onion, chilies, etcetera. **Variant:** flour, ground walnut, chopped onion, egg, oil, salt and water. |

## For coating without using egg:

| Ingredients | Preparation |
|---|---|
| ½ cup of chickpea flour<br>½ cup of wheat flour<br>¼ cup of wheat germ<br>3 tbs. of onion<br>2 tsp. of nutmeg<br>1 tsp. baking powder<br>2 tbs. of oil<br>Sea salt to taste<br>Warm water as needed | Blend all ingredients until achieving a consistency of thick atole (cornmeal gruel). |

## Crepes (basic recipe)

| Ingredients | Preparation |
|---|---|
| 1 cup of flour<br>3 tbs. of olive oil<br>3 eggs<br>½ tsp of salt<br>Cow's or soy milk as necessary | Place all ingredients in the bowl of an electric blender; beat thoroughly and add milk until obtaining a liquid mixture. Refrigerate for 6 hours or overnight.<br>Spread a little oil in a small pan (only use oil for in the first crepe), add a tbs. of paste and move the pan quickly to spread paste and form a thin layer, or spread paste with a spoon. Cook both sides. If you are not going to eat the crepes straightaway, allow to cool, wrap in wax paper and refrigerate. They can be preserved for several days. You can make 30 thin crepes using a small pan; they must be soft.<br>These crepes can be used for both savory and sweet dishes. |

# Pecan and mushroom pâté

| Ingredients | Preparation |
|---|---|
| 300 grams of thinly sliced mushrooms<br>100 grams of finely chopped pecans<br>1½ chopped onion,<br>1 chopped large clove of garlic<br>Olive oil<br>Sea salt to taste | Wash the mushrooms. Sauté garlic and onion in a pan in a little oil; add mushrooms and salt and cook for 10-15 minutes. Add walnuts. Refrigerate until served. |

# Mushroom pate

| Ingredients | Preparation |
|---|---|
| ¼ kilo of chopped mushrooms,<br>½ small chopped onion<br>½ lime (juice)<br>2 tbs. of breadcrumbs<br>Oregano and parsley to taste | Wash mushrooms well. Sauté onion, add mushrooms and remaining ingredients. Blend all together in a little water and add breadcrumbs slowly until achieving the desired consistency. |

# Olive pâté

| Ingredients | Preparation |
|---|---|
| 1 jar of seedless black olives<br>1 small clove of garlic<br>¼ tsp. of cumin powder<br>2 tbs. of olive oil | Drain olives well. Blend all ingredients until obtaining a paste. Serve on tostadas or Havana style cookies. |

## Pecan pâté

| Ingredients | Preparation |
|---|---|
| 300　grams of peeled pecans<br>½tbs. of miso or<br>2tbs. of tahini<br>　Water as needed | Blend ingredients well until achieving a texture similar to that of pâté.<br>Tahini is the paste of sesame seeds.<br>Miso is a by-product of the fermentation soy or other cereals– you may find it in stores selling Chinese products. |

## Eggplant pâté

| Ingredients | Preparation |
|---|---|
| 1　eggplant<br>½　small red onion<br>2　cloves of garlic<br>2　tbs. of tahini (sesame seed paste)<br>1　lime (juice)<br>　Olive oil as necessary<br>　Sea salt to taste<br>　Cumin, parsley and coriander to taste | Fry eggplant in olive oil and a little salt.<br>Blend all ingredients. |

## Tofu cream

| Ingredients | Preparation |
|---|---|
| 2　cups of tofu<br>1　lime (juice)<br>¼　tsp. of grated ginger<br>3　tbs. of virgin olive oil<br>　Sea salt to taste | Blend all ingredients and then place in a bain-marie for 15 minutes.<br>If you like a more intense flavor, add seaweed.<br>You can spread tofu, cream on sandwiches, pizzas, etcetera. |

## Veganesa (mayonnaise without egg)

| Ingredients | Preparation |
|---|---|
| 1　cup of virgin olive oil<br>⅓　cup of soy milk<br>½　clove of garlic<br>½　lime (juice)<br>　Sea salt to taste | Blend all ingredients until well mixed.<br>You can make colored sauces by adding cooked carrot (orange); beetroot (pink); avocado (green); mustard (yellow) or fried tomato (red). |

## Vegan ranch dressing

| Ingredients | Preparation |
|---|---|
| ½ cup mayonnaise | Mix all the ingredients in a blender and |
| ½ cup veganaise | blend until smooth and creamy. |
| ¼ cup soy milk | Transfer to a storage container with lid |
| ½ tsp garlic salt | and refrigerate until use. |
| ½ tsp garlic powder | |
| ½ tsp onion powder | |
| ¼ tsp white pepper | |
| 2 tsp fresh parsley, chopped | |
| 1 ½ cider vinegar | |
| ½ tsp dill | |

## Brown gravy

| Ingredients | Preparation |
|---|---|
| 1 Tbsp corn starch | Mix corn starch, soy sauce and vegetable |
| 2 Tbsp soy sauce | seasoning together in sauce pan. |
| ½ tsp vegetable seasoning | Gradually add water, stir well. |
| 2 cups water | Cook over moderate heat until thick. |
| ¼ tahini (sesame butter) | Add tahini. Mix well |

## Guacamole

| Ingredients | Preparation |
|---|---|
| 2 ripe avocados | Peel avocados and mash; add onion, tomato, |
| 1 finely chopped red tomato | chilies, lime juice and salt. Mix well. |
| ¼ finely chopped onion | Serve on tostadas or bread, or as a garnish. |
| 2 finely chopped Serrano chilies | |
| ½ lime (juice) | |
| Sea salt to taste | |

## Potato tortilla (without egg)

Preparation:
Fry finely diced potatoes in very hot olive oil (you may add chopped onion, red or green pepper, leek or Mexican squash to obtain a juicier tortilla).
While frying, prepare the egg substitute, which consists of a mixture of chickpea flour, water, and a little salt and pepper. Mix with a fork until achieving a creamy texture, without lumps (the amount depends on the potatoes used). When the potatoes are fried, remove from heat, drain oil and mix potatoes with dough. Leave a little oil in the pan at a low heat, pour in the mixture and move the pan to avoid sticking. When one side is cooked, turn it over and cook the other side. Allow to cool before serving so that it does not break up.

## Mash potatoes

| Ingredients | Preparation |
| --- | --- |
| 8 potatoes | Place potatoes in a large pot and cover with |
| 3 cloves garlic, roasted | water; add 3 tsp of salt. Bring to a boil and |
| ¾ cup chives, chopped | cook for 15 minutes or until potatoes are |
| 3 Tbsp dairy-free margarine | soft; drain and transfer to a large bowl. |
| 3 Tbsp rosemary | Add roasted garlic, margarine, and 1 cup |
| 1 cup vegetable broth | vegetable broth; mach or blend; add more |
| Sea salt and pepper to taste | broth for desired consistency. Add chives, |
| | rosemary, salt an pepper to taste. |

## Croutons

| Ingredients | Preparation |
| --- | --- |
| 2 cups bread, cubed | Preheat oven to 350o F. |
| 1 Tbsp fresh thyme leaves, chopped | Combine all crouton ingredients together. |
| 1 Tbsp olive oil | Bake until golden brown, about 10-15 |
| Pinch ground black pepper or to taste | minutes. Let to cool. |

# Alternative Dishes

## SUGGESTIONS TO PLAN YOUR MENUS:

- Take in consideration the flavor and the aspect of your meals, because we eat with the eyes first, which are the ones that stimulate our appetite.

- Combine dishes that require different cooking methods.

- Have a variety of sauces that are served in the same meal.

- Eat balanced and nutritious food.

- Consider side dishes a great support to entrees; they can also be served as the main course.

- Know that there are more than 4,000 vegetarian dishes among which you can choose, and combine them.

## VEGETABLE BROTH

Use this method to extract the most flavor from the vegetables.
8 cups water and vegetables like: carrot, onion, garlic, potato, fennel, fresh herbs, ginger, washed organic vegetable skins, leek green and white parts, soy sauce, etcetera.
Bring to boil (low heat), partially covered 45-60 minutes.
Strain into a clean pot or heat proof plastic container, pressing down on the vegetables to extract the juices.
Let cool, uncovered, then refrigerate until ready to use.

## BROWN RICE

Use 2 ¼ cups brown rice to 2 ½ cups water for long grain or
2 to 2 ¼ water for short grain brown rice
Bring to boil in a saucepan:
2 ½ cups water and
1 tbsp. olive oil
½ tsp sea salt or to taste
Add and stir 1 cup brown rice
Cover and cook over very low heat until all water is absorbed (40-45 minutes).
Do not lift the lid before the end of cooking. Let stand covered for a few minutes before serving.

# CRUNCHY VEGETABLE

4 tbsp. nondairy cream cheese (try tofutti brand)
4 pitas cut in half
1 cup fresh spinach, shredded
½ cup red cabbage, shredded
¼ cup alfalfa sprouts
½ cup fresh tomatoes, chopped
½ cup avocado, sliced
½ cup cucumbers, diced
2 tbsp. red onion, finely diced and Sea salt to taste
Spread 1 tablespoon of cream cheese over each half pita. Sprinkle an even amount of the remaining ingredients in each half pita. Serve.

# TOFU OMELET

1 packet firm tofu, drained
2-3 Tbsp nutritional yeast
1 Tbsp tahini butter
1 Tbsp tamari or salt
1 Tbsp safflower oil
Mash all ingredients, except oil.
In a medium skillet, heat oil over medium heat, spoon batter into skillet and form into an omelet shape. Cook until underside is browned. Flip and cook other side. Serve hot.
Variations: for scrambled, simply scramble the batter. If you want, stir in cooked diced onion and bell pepper into batter before cooking.

# SOYBEAN BURGERS

3 cups soybeans, cooked and drained
¼ cup tamari
¼ cup sunflower oil
¼ tsp ground cayenne
2 cloves garlic, minced
½ cup carrots, grated
½ green bell pepper, finely chopped
1 celery stalk, finely chopped
1 ½ cups millet, cooked
2 cups quick (not instant) rolled oats
Additional light oil for browning
In a food processor, combine soybeans, tamari, oil, cayenne, and garlic. Process until smooth, then transfer to large mixing bowl.
Stir in remaining ingredients (except additional oil) mixing well.
In a large skillet, heat thin layer of oil over medium-high heat. Scoop out amount of bean mixture and shape into a patty (wet hands as necessary so they don't stick) and place each patty into hot oil. Brown on one side then turn and brown other side 2-3 minutes.
Repeat with remaining mixture.

## PIZZA TOPPINGS

Pizza toppings are limited only by your imagination. Some ideas:
- Try soy Parmesan cheese or nutritional yeast
- Add different sauces like red pepper, garlic puree, or any kind of pesto
- Veggies that you have available and drizzle some crushed tomatoes over them.
- For Mexican, try refried beans, tomatoes, soy cheese and salsa
- Try fake meats, top with veggie burger crumbles or veggie bacon, or veggie pepperoni.
- Try with tofu, sun dried tomatoes, beans, spinach or even corn.

# Sandwiches, Easy Snacks And Appetizers

**Sandwich fillings can be just about anything you have available.**
- Fill a bagel with tofu cream cheese with olives or veggie salami, avocado and onion.
- Fill a baguette with lettuce, tomato, veggie turkey and nondairy cheese slices.
- Fill a pita bread with faux tuna or 'chicken' salad (try Worthington's or Chicketts products, mixed with vegan mayo and celery.
- Fill whole wheat bread with soy cheese, avocado, onion, sprouts, etcetera.
- Heat sliced veggie dogs and vegetarian style baked beans in the microwave.
- Hot tortillas, fill with refried beans, salsa, guacamole and corn for easy burritos.
- Pasta salad: mix cooked spiral pasta either chopped broccoli, carrots, green pepper, corn, red onion and your favorite vinaigrette.
- Zap a veggie burger in microwave. Put it on a bun with your favorite condiments.

**Appetizers can be as simple as dip and chips or vegetarian pâté:**
- Mix for a Mexican dip using refried beans, green olives, salsa, shredded soy cheese, tofutti sour cream, sliced yellow onions and jalapeños.
- Bake bite-size pieces of mock 'chicken' or tofu and serve with toothpicks.
- Try fish-free vegan caviar. Looks, just like the red thing.
- Try using tofu and vegetarian hot dogs wrapped in puff pastry.

## STEAMED VEGETABLES

Steam all desired vegetables that you have available.
E.g.: carrots, cabbage, zucchini, onion, broccoli, potato, sweet potato, red bell pepper, cauliflower, artichoke hearts, etcetera. Serve with main dish.

## EGGS SUBSTITUTION

| Non sweet preparation options: | Sweet preparation options: |
|---|---|
| Battered eggs can be substituted for: <br> * Chickpea flour with wheat flour. <br> - Special flour for breading <br> - Cooking flour with no eggs <br> - Tempura flour <br> - Soybean flour dissolved in water "four teaspoons of water for every two teaspoons of flour for every egg you want to substitute". <br> - Two teaspoons of ground flax seed dissolved in four teaspoons of water | In cakes, pies, crepes, biscuits,…they can be substituted for: <br> - Special flour for cooking with no eggs. <br> - Soybean flour dissolve in water "four teaspoons of water for every two teaspoons of flour for every egg you want to substitute". <br> - A very ripe mashed banana (you can use cantaloupe, pear, apple). <br> - Two teaspoons of ground flax seed dissolved in four teaspoons of water |

# Guide For A Vegetarian
# New Terms Used In This Book

(This guide is taken from: Compassion over killing's Vegetarian Starter Guide and Vegetarian Times)

## Tofu

It is white, easily digested. Use in Asian cooking, is a high-protein soybean product. Tofu comes in many different textures and rapidly absorbs flavors and spices. Use it in scrambled with nutritional yeast and other seasonings in place of eggs, or in stir-fries or marinate or bake it as an entrée; for dressings, shakes, and pie and dessert fillings.

## Nutritional yeast

It is a dietary supplement and a condiment that has a distinct but pleasant aroma. This product is inactive yeast rich in vitamins and minerals, with delicious cheesy flavor. It can be added to soups, casseroles, stews or to make any dish creamier or sprinkled on toast, popcorn or spaghetti. It will be a pleasant surprise.

## Soy cheese

It is a non-dairy cheese made from soybeans. Use it as a cheese substitute in any dish you decided. Check the product label as some brands contain casein, a cow's milk protein.

## Soy margarine

It is a tasty, non-dairy version of butter without the cholesterol (and cruelty) found in other butters and margarines.

## TVP (textured vegetable protein)

It is a dried soy product and a simple substitute for ground beef in stews, chili, and pasta sauce.

## Seitan or gluten

Also known as wheat meat is a delicious, high-protein meat substitute. Made primarily from wheat gluten, find it prepackaged in a variety of flavors and dishes. Try seitan in your favorite entrée recipe or in a stir-fry, casseroles, stews, and etcetera.

## Soy and rice milks

They are healthy alternatives to cow's milk. Increasingly available in your local grocery store (as well as in health food stores), soy or rice milk come in flavors. Try it on your favorite cereal, in your coffee or drink it straight, or in any recipe that calls for milk. Each of the dozens of brands of soy and rice milks has its own distinct taste, so taste test to find the one you like best.

### Ener-G's Egg replacer

It is a ready-made product available in most health food stores that is not only quick and easy to use when recipes call for eggs as a binding agent (such as in baking), but is also cholesterol-free.

## Miso

A salty paste made from cooked, aged soybeans and sometimes grains. Thick and spreadable, it's also used for flavoring soup bases. Available in several varieties; darker varieties tend to be stronger flavored and saltier than lighter varieties.

## Tamari

It is a naturally brewed soy sauce that contains no sugar. Wheat-free.

## Umeboshi plum paste

A condiment made from Japanese sour plums that are salted, sun-dried and aged. This contains iron, calcium, minerals, vitamin C, and enzymes.

## Saffron

A spice derived from the autumn crocus. It has a yellow color and distinctive taste.

## Shallot

This is a small, mild-flavored onion like bulb. It is between garlic and onion.

## Dijon mustard

French-style smooth mustard made with mustard seed, white wine and seasonings.

## Sesame oil

Extracted from sesame seeds, it comes in two basic types, light and dark. Lighter varieties are good for salad dressings and sautés; dark in traditional Japanese cuisine.

## Nori

It is rich in protein, calcium, vitamins, iron, and minerals. Crispy sheets of pressed sea vegetable. Used for Japanese sushi rolled around rice or crumbled as a garnish.

# Desserts

## CHOCOLATE PUDDING

| 1 ½ cups soy or rice milk<br>¼ cup cocoa powder<br>¼ maple syrup<br>¼ tsp vanilla extract<br>3 Tbsp cornstarch | Mix all the ingredients except vanilla.<br>Once the mixture is smooth, cook over medium heat, stirring constantly until the pudding thickens.<br>Stir in the vanilla and mix well. Pour into individual serving dishes.<br>Refrigerate until chilled and serve |

## CHOCOLATE MOUSE

| 1 ¼ lbs. tofu<br>¾ cup chocolate chips, melted. | In a blender, purée the tofu to a smooth paste. Add the melted chocolate and blend thoroughly. Pour the mousse into individual serving dishes, chilled and serve. |

## STRAWBERRY MANGO CRISP

| 4 cups quartered strawberries<br>2 cups mango, diced<br>4 tbsp. brown sugar<br>4 tbsp. flour<br>Toping:<br>1 cup flour<br>½ cup rolled oats<br>1 cup brown sugar<br>½ cup (1 stick) soy margarine | Preheat oven at 400o F<br>Mix the first four ingredients together. Place into a 2quart casserole dish. Set aside.<br>Mix the dry ingredients together in a medium bowl. Cut in the margarine until the mixture resembles small peas. Spread the topping evenly over the fruit mixture.<br>Bake for 35-45 minutes, until bubbly.<br>Serve warm with nondairy 'ice cream'. |

## APPLE PIE

| 8 apples, cut in thinly sliced<br>1 tbsp. lemon juice<br>4 tbsp. applesauce<br>¾ cup brown sugar<br>1 tbsp. cinnamon<br>¼ tsp nutmeg<br>1/8 tsp sea salt<br>2 tbsp. soy margarine<br>2 tbsp. flour<br>2 pastry crust for 9' pie | Line bottom of pan with one-half of rolled pastry.<br>Mix apples with lemon juice.<br>Combine sugar, cinnamon, nutmeg, flour, apple purée, salt and add to the apples slices.<br>Fill the pastry shell with the apple mixture.<br>Dot evenly with the margarine.<br>Cover apples with remaining half of pastry and bake at 450o F for 10 minutes. reduce heat to 350o F and bake about 40 minutes.<br>Serve warm. |

## TOFU PUMPKIN PIE

| | |
|---|---|
| 2 cups pumpkin purée<br>1 ½ cups firm tofu, drained<br>¼ tsp ground nutmeg<br>1 tsp ground cinnamon<br>¼ tsp ground ginger<br>¼ tsp ground cloves<br>¼ tsp ground allspice<br>2 tsp pumpkin pie spice<br>¼ cup cornstarch<br>½ tsp sea salt<br>1 cup light brown sugar<br>4 Tbsp vegetable oil<br>2 tsp vanilla extract<br>Unbaked pie crust | Preheat oven to 350o F<br>Combine all fillings ingredients in a blender.<br>Process until smooth<br>Add ¼ tsp of ginger.<br>Pour filling into crust.<br>Bake 60 minutes. Let cool.<br>**Note**: you can replace pumpkin for squash |

## SWEET POTATO PIE

| | |
|---|---|
| 4 cups sweet potato, mashed<br>2 Tbsp soy margarine<br>2 cups soymilk or rice milk<br>1 cup light brown sugar or to taste<br>2 tsp molasses<br>1 tsp almond extract<br>1 tsp vanilla extract<br>2 tsp cinnamon<br>1 tsp sea salt<br>½ tsp nutmeg<br>½ tsp ground ginger<br>¼ tsp cardamom<br>1 tbsp. tapioca flour<br>2 prepared pie shells | In a food processor, mix all the ingredients slowly until everything is combined. Then mix on high for a few minutes and pulse until mostly smooth.<br>Bake 2 pie shells for 7 minutes at 400o F.<br>Fill shells all the ways to the top and bake at 400o F for 1 hour.<br>Pies should not jiggle very much when you take them out of the oven. If this happens you will need to bake a little longer until they are slightly firm.<br>Let them cool then cover and refrigerate to chill before serving. |

# SWEET POTATO BAKE

| | |
|---|---|
| 4 medium sweet potatoes, peeled, cooked<br>½ cup fresh orange juice<br>Dash sea salt<br>1 tsp ginger powder<br>½ tsp cinnamon<br>Dash nutmeg<br>½ cup pecans, chopped<br>1/3 cup light brown sugar<br>¼ cup unbleached flour<br>2 tbsp. soy margarine | Mash sweet potatoes with orange juice, ginger and salt. Spoon into deep baking pan.<br>Mix well flour, pecans, sugar and margarine.<br>Spoon pecan mixture over the sweet potatoes.<br>Sprinkle the top with cinnamon and nutmeg.<br>Bake at 350o F for 25 minutes. |

# A Glance At Enzymes

The wisdom of nature
can overcome all the
possibilities of Science.
**Nietzsche.**

Enzymes are the effective key of the principle of intangible life of the magnetic energy in the Cosmos. Dr. Norman W. Walker.

VITAL PRINCIPLE - ATOMS - MOLECULES - ENZYMES.

The secret of always feeling healthy may be found in our own body. Nature has created a magical healing power in each cell, tissue, gland, and organ, and in the organism's metabolic process: the enzymes. Enzymes are complex protein-based biological substances that are found in all living cells, either vegetable or animal, and they have an influence on all our physical and mental functions. We need the life force of enzymes to have a healthy mind and body.

These complex substances (soluble chemical-organic substances) are intangible elements (electrical-magnetic), found in natural food such as seeds, bean sprouts, fruits and raw vegetables that nourish the body (cells and tissues) and that function as catalyzers (metabolic activators), in other words, they do not undergo any change, catalyze the chemical action of atoms and molecules causing a transformed reaction in the metabolic process, working quickly at body temperature. Enzymes enable us to digest food and absorb nutrients that provide life and health.

When we eat fresh and raw food, our cells produce new enzymes that destroy free radicals, and improve their built-in protective enzyme system (induction of enzymes). Cooking at high temperature ($54^{0C}$) kills enzymes, in addition to which if the pH (acid/base balance) changes, it affects the enzymatic activity of the organism. Less digestive enzymes are produced as we get older. If the digestive system has insufficient enzymes, the amount of toxins in the colon increases, leading to tumors, ulcers, etc.

The ASE suffix indicates the enzymes and the substrate that causes the action.

Example:  saccharose  +  saccharase  =  glucose + fructose  +  saccharase

(substrate) - (enzyme)  =  (products)  -  (enzyme)

Example: honey contains the following enzymes: invertase (a tonic against intestinal slowness); amylase (effective for intestinal peristaltic movement), and catalase (the alcoholic detoxifying power of honey).

Enzymes play a role in digestion, breathing, photosynthesis, coagulation of the blood, the chemistry of sight, and the synthesis of proteins.

Where are enzymes found?

Our body creates many enzymes from substances such as food, liquid and air. Nutrients help to stimulate the vigor of enzymes.

There are over 700 different types of enzymes, each of which has a specific function. One turns food into energy, another turns it into carbohydrates, another turns it into protein, and turn it into various vitamins and minerals, fat, etc. Each cellular reaction depends on the biological response commenced and controlled by a specific system of enzymes.

All enzymes are vital. Following is a list of twelve enzymes and their invigorating functions:

1) Ptyalin is found in the saliva glands of the mouth. It acts on carbohydrates and starch. It creates a form of dextrin and maltose and it produces energy.

2) Pepsin is found in the digestive system. It acts on food containing protein. It produces amino acids such as peptones and proteose that are used for circulation of the blood, the bones, glands, cells and tissues to nourish and rebuild the organism

3) Chymosin is found in the digestive system and acts on dairy products. It facilitates coagulation and changes casein (a milk protein) in amino-acids. It metabolizes milk minerals (casein, calcium, phosphorous and magnesium) and sends them to the blood flow in order to facilitate invigoration of the bones, teeth and arterial neural systems.

4) Lipase is found in the digestive system. It acts on the fats of dairy products and transports-stores vitamins and minerals.

5) Trypsin is found in the intestinal-pancreas region. It carries on the digestive function of dairy products, such as extracting amino acids from proteins, vitamins and minerals so that they may be used by the cells, tissues and organs of the entire body.

6) Steapsin is found in the intestines. It acts on the fats of dairy products and metabolizes fats and turns them into essential fatty acids that are used to lubricate the arteries and keep the blood flow healthy.

7) Amylopsin is found in the intestines. It acts on the assimilation of the starch found in nutrients and produces a glucose-energy sub-product.

8) Invertase is found in the intestines. It acts on the sugars found in nutrients, facilitates the metabolism of natural sugars and produces forms of glucose and fructose that are

160

stored in the organs, so that they are available as sources of energy for the body and for the thinking process.

9) Maltose is found in the intestines. It acts on cereals and bread and facilitates the conversion of carbohydrates digested by ptyalin to produce maltose that, in turn, creates dextrin, in other words, natural sugar that produces energy.

10) Lactose is found in the intestines. It acts on the sugar found in dairy products and facilitates the conversion of sugar into glucose and galactose both of which are used to produce energy and vitality.

11) Hydrochloric acid is found in the intestinal-digestive system. It acts on heavy proteins and extracts amino acids into the blood flow in order to give the organism energy. It boosts vitamins and minerals so that they may carry out their functions properly.

12) Erepsin is found in the intestines. It acts on the proteins and peptides found in nutrients. It turns proteins into useful amino-acids in order to regenerate the entire organism, both internally and externally.

# A Glance At Fats

You do not have anything if you do not digest properly
**Voltaire.**

Fat is the most concentrated source of energy there is. It complements glucides and protides that consume less oxygen than fat and whose muscular performance is high, although they have a different biological value. Insufficient fat causes renal alterations and other health problems. Fats provide a valuable quantity of calories. The perfect balance of calories in our body is 30% originating from fat. Fats are indispensable, particularly for the heart and cells. Prostaglandins are produced inside each cell of the organism and regulate many of its functions. Prostaglandins are formed from essential oils.

The lipoids of oils and fats contain some lypo-soluble vitamins (A, D, E and K). Fat helps to absorb calcium and balance the body's level of cholesterol, and are used to form sexual hormones. In order to maintain a healthy and balanced diet, you should correctly select the type of fats you wish to consume (that should be of different origin), the quantity of which depends on the weather conditions, type of work (physical or intellectual), what type of sport you indulge in, amount of activity, etc. Consuming fat in large quantities causes problems such as acne, blackheads, greasy skin, aging and overweight (obesity and malnutrition may be related). If you maintain a balanced diet you need not worry about the quantities you take on.

Fats are divided into three categories:

Saturated fat = lard (white animal fat) and butter.

Monounsaturated fat = olive oil

Polyunsaturated fat = corn oil (omega 6) safflower oil and sunflower oil.

Unsaturated fatty acids should be eaten with meals but only in small quantities. Fat may accumulate in the body in large quantities in the form of small drops of intracellular fat that is used as a reserve, a source of heat and energy during times of fasting, when it is cold, etc.

Polyunsaturated fats are the most recommended as they maintain a balance between Omega-3 and Omega-6 (soy milk, linseed and canola). Take Omega-3 (alpha-linoleic acid, 2 grams a day) is found in seaweed in abundance, as well as in green plants (purslane), oleaginous products and flaxseed. Deficiency of Omega-3 in the body leads to reduced sight both in the brain and in the retina. Omega-6 (linoleic acid, 2 grams a day) is found in soy bean oil, corn oil, black raisin seeds, sunflower seeds and other vegetable oils, such as milk, butter and animal fat.

DHA (decosahexanoic acid) is an important polyunsaturated fat for the brain and the eyes. It is an excellent source of nutrition, a pre-hormone considered as the gene-enzyme that regulates age, metabolism and prevents cancerous tumors.

The word "oil" originates from the world "olive". Vegetable oils (corn, sunflower, soy, olive, etc.) are easy to assimilate and contain unsaturated fats that are the most suitable for our body. Vegetable fat, such as that found in oleaginous products (nuts, almonds, etc.) and seeds, grain, cereals, olives and avocado, should be consumed naturally.

Oils are not nutrients; they just provide calories and energy. Heating oils to a high temperature (frying) alters their molecular structure, makes them indigestible and toxic for the body. Frequent consumption causes arteriosclerosis and constitutes a slow and shameful means of suicide. "Burnt" oil produces a powerful poison called butyric acid.

Animal fats are saturated fats and include lard (removed from the fat of pigs), tallow (hard and solid animal fat) and bacon, the fatty meat of pigs. Cacao and coconut are also saturated fats. Saturated fats block linoleic acid (Omega-6). Linoleic acid changes when it is fried or processed.

# A Glance At Carbohydrates

The human body is a slave of the mind…
and also of the spirit. If you wish to have healthy
body you must keep alive your desire to have one.
**Dr. Bernard Jensen.**

Plants extract water from the soil and carbon dioxide from the air and the sun's energy joins these two elements, thus forming complex chains called sugars or starches. All plants contain starch, protein, fat, vitamins, minerals and fiber.

Carbohydrates are the most essential aspect of human nutrition. Their function is to regulate the internal secretion of glands. Carbohydrates or carbon hydrates are sugar and starch based that, together with fat, provide the main source of heat and energy. If we do not take exercise to convert this source of heat, then it turns into a reserve and, subsequently, obesity. When there is sufficient combustion of glucose (sugars), fatty bodies are burned by the organism, however, insufficient combustion produces residue that lodges in the tissues. This residue turns into starch that eventually leads to illness. If we lead a sedentary way of life, the consumption of sugar is reduced to a minimum.

Consumption of glucose should represent 55% of our total daily intake of calories; fats 30% and protein 15%. When there is insufficient glucose, fat and proteins replace it, and also create a sensation of hunger. Each gram of glucose provides 4 calories. Carbohydrates or sugars are obtained from most types of food, such as flour, bread, vegetables and dry and fresh fruit, which may be directly assimilated and help to rebuild tissues. Starches and sugars are forms of carbohydrates that nourish the body so that it may perform its physical and muscular activities.

The most recommendable source of starches include whole meal cereals, seeds, bananas, and root vegetables, such as sweet potato, yucca and potatoes. The most recommendable sugars are molasses, which have a high content of nutrients, bee's honey and maguey honey.

Do not make whole meal bread with lard and eggs, as these make it a very difficult type of food for the organism to assimilate. If the paper bag is impregnated with fat when you buy bread, do not eat the bread.

White sugar provides "empty" calories that do not contain any nutrients. The organism needs vitamins and minerals in order to metabolize white sugar. After consuming white sugar, a considerable amount of calcium is lost through urine and there is a major reduction in phosphorous (phosphorous is essential for providing energy for the body and thinking) in the blood to the detriment of the osseous system. Calcium, phosphorous and magnesium are balanced against one another in the body. Industrial sugars irritate mucus, ferment in the intestine, damage the digestive organs, overload the liver and pancreas, and cause constipation and decalcification.

# A Glance At Proteins

A simple diet makes life cheaper,
prevents illness, improves health,
keeps the mind clear and makes you
a more suitable person to provide an
efficient service.
**Dr. Rossiter.**

Proteins contain the basic material of life. The four basic essential elements for living things are oxygen, nitrogen, hydrogen and carbon, as well as sulfur, phosphorous, iron, copper and zinc, depending on their function, the amount of the elements.

Protides (proteins, albumin = nitrogenous elements) are very complex organic compounds formed by a group of amino acids that the body needs to return it to its normal condition. A protein molecule contains 23 different amino acids, 15 of which are produced by the body and 8 (essential) must be included as part of our daily diet (fruit, vegetables, oleaginous products, seeds, bean sprouts and grain). When amino acids enter the blood flow, they are transported throughout the entire body to build, repair and preserve cells and tissues and provide the blood the purity it needs.

When the organism takes on complete protein, it breaks it down into amino acids in order to form the proteins that the body needs. When the body needs amino acids, it obtains them from the blood system, the lymphatic system, the liver and from cells (that releases them from the blood), or wherever there are protein reserves. The organism "recycles" 70% of protein, more or less 20% of total body weight.

Proteins are essential: they form the structure of the organism and enable human beings to grow and develop. They form the bones, skin, nails, hair, muscles, the heart and blood. Proteins do not produce energy, they consume it!

The right amount of protein depends on age, weight, sex, weather, activity (physical or intellectual, etc), however, in general terms, one gram of protein for each kilogram of body weight on the natural basis of stature, etc (not weight).

Proteins play an active role in a wide range of vital processes in the thousands of millions of cells of the muscles and various organs, and they are constantly dying and being reborn. They are involved in the building of tissues, balancing liquids and help to assimilate food, intensify the metabolism and have the principles of construction and fixing. They are cellular stimulants, act on the acid/mineral salt base, antibodies, enzymes, hormones, genetic transmission and structures. When the body has excess proteins, it excretes a part and it turns the other into glucose or fat for storage. Fat delays the digestion of protein. Excess protein is turned into toxic and acid elements (nitric, lactic, etc.), leading to illness of the organism and the strain in balance themselves result in tissues and food conceding their alkaline salts. Excess toxic acids causes edema, overweight, cellulites, gray hair, baldness, dark circle under the eyes, nervousness and premature wrinkles on the face.

Insufficient proteins affect the sensibility and coordination of movement, or break the balance of liquids with accumulation in the interstitial space of cells. Another consequence is that the organism begins to "eat" its own tissue (skin, muscles), so they become weak and are consumed (aging) to give the brain, heart and lungs what they require.

A complete protein is simply obtained from 2/3 of cereal and 1/3 of legumes (the amino acids missing in cereals are provided by legumes), for example: 2/3 corn and 1/3 beans = one complete protein. The combination of legumes and cereal includes minerals, vitamins, carbohydrates, fats and fiber.

In order to obtain all the proteins you need you should combine:

a) Cereals with legumes.

b) Dairy products with legumes.

c) Dairy products with cereals.

d) Dairy products with oleaginous products and seeds.

If eating legumes produces gas in the intestine, eat less until your intestinal tract has adjusted itself. Soaking beans (or any legumes) overnight before cooking makes digestion easier.

Sources of protein: Dairy products, egg yolk, oleaginous products, legumes, cereals and fruit. Lentils and soy beans contain complete protein.

The following foods contain amino acids that the body does not produce: carrots, bananas, Brussels sprouts, cabbage, cauliflower, corn, cucumber, eggplant, peas, potatoes, red tomatoes and pumpkin. Oleaginous products include: sesame seeds, sunflower seeds and peanuts (eat just a few as they are a form of concentrated protein).

# A Glance At Vitamins

"The powerful life forces that create and develop trees and vitamins,
condensed into high quantities in the fruits of these trees,
may not be calculated in calories or
in vulgar chemical materials".
**Dr. Paul Carton.**

Vitamins are essential elements for life (in Latin *vita*=life). They are perishable organic substances that are found in natural foods in variable quantities. Our body needs them in small amounts and each vitamin plays an important role in the body's metabolism.

Vitamins do not provide the body energy; they fix other nutrients, although they are needed for the functioning of the body and for using and storing energy, activating oxidation of food, and metabolic functions. They help to form tissue. They play a major role in our metabolism and insufficient vitamins may cause various and serious alterations. We obtain vitamins from raw food such as fresh fruit (also in juices), vegetables (in salads) and oleaginous products (nuts, almonds, pine nuts, etc.)

There are two types of vitamins: hydro-soluble (soluble in water) that must be replaced daily, examples being vitamin C and complex B, and lypo-soluble vitamins (soluble in fat) that are stored in adipose tissues and the liver and remain in the body longer, examples being vitamins A, D, E and K. Too many lypo-soluble vitamins may intoxicate the body as they are not easily excreted. Excess hydro-soluble vitamins are excreted in urine, sweat and feces.

Anti-oxidant vitamins include A, E and C (garlic, onion and avocado) and selenium. Caffeine, alcohol and cigarettes (a cigarette consumes 25 mg of vitamin C) produce a high level of oxidation. If you believe you are lacking any vitamins, eat food that contains them in order to balance your bodily requirements. Insufficient vitamins, minerals or nutrients cause many problems so therapy with large doses taken under medical supervision is recommended so as to produce visible results.

## Bioflavonoid

All natural foods contain bioflavonoid, some of which replace vitamins E and C. They are anti-oxidants, of which there is a wide variety, over 500. They survive at high temperature. The bioflavonoid called pycnogenol is a powerful protective supplement obtained from the bark and leaves of pine trees.

**What are anti-oxidants?** Anti-oxidants are a source of vitality and health. Free radicals are non-neutralized micro-particles that make other molecules to recover electrons that are missing, damaging, and altering molecules of carbohydrates, proteins, fats, DNA and RNA, changing their structure and function.

Anti-oxidants neutralize the action of free radicals, giving part of their electrons and thus delaying the aging process and destruction of cells. Having the correct level of anti-oxidants protects us against cardiovascular disease and various types of cancer.

**Anti-oxidants are found in fruit and vegetables** such as cabbage, spinach, carrots, potatoes, parsley, melon, egg yolk (B12) and dairy products, all of which are high in vitamin A, and limes, oranges, bananas, pears, papaya, green pepper, strawberries, pineapples and red tomatoes, rich in vitamin C. They are also found in whole meal cereals, peanuts, vegetable oils, oleaginous products, wheat germ, rice and yeast. Food that contains zinc includes milk, pumpkin seeds and sunflower seeds.

With this variety we can combine and prepare very nutritional dishes and salads and take on a reasonable quantity of anti-oxidants.

Biological fuel for the cells: vitamins, minerals, amino acids and trace elements.

Do you know how vitamins help the organism?

## Vitamin A (Retinol)

This is associated with sight, growth, formation of bones, formation and conservation of the skin, setting up defenses, and reproduction.

Fats and minerals are required for it to be assimilated. It acts as an anti-oxidant on cells and eliminates free radicals. These molecules are unbalanced because atoms have lost an electron. They constitute super oxides or ultraviolet light that kill part of the living cell through oxidizing destruction. If it affects the nucleus of genetic material it could change and may produce a pre-cancerous cell. It is essential for the tissues, including ocular tissue (myopia, night blindness), during pregnancy and breast feeding, helps to prevent allergies, acne, dry skin, asthma, catarrh, emphysema, colitis, hyperthyroidism, diabetes and rheumatism, and also aids the proper functioning of the immunity system. It keeps the skin, hair, gums and teeth healthy and protects smokers' lungs.

Ninety percent of vitamin A is stored in the liver, as well as in the eyes, blood, kidneys, lungs and fatty tissues. The body uses reserves when it is tense if a diet does not include sufficient vitamin A. When children consume too much vitamin A, their bones become fragile (tending to fracture), whereas in women it results in abnormal development of the fetus. The body converts beta-carotene into Vitamin A, although only the amount it needs. Every day you need 15 mg of carotene (you should consume up to 60 mg). A thousand units of vitamin A = 6 mg of carotene and one carrot has 12 mg of beta-carotene. Beta-carotene protects the organism's cells against sunlight, oxidizing agents and free radicals, and helps to prevent burns and skin cancer. Carotene pigment may be found in roots, stems, flowers and fruits.

**Vitamin A helps** to create enzymes in the liver, promote growth of the body and its harmonious development, improve appetite and digestion, form membranes and tissues and maintain the normal function of the skin, mucus and night vision. It helps the immunity system, has protective properties and provides resistance to infections and parasites. It also prevents problems of the bladder, mouth, esophagus, the gastrointestinal system and the lungs.

**Problems caused by deficiency:** night blindness, red eyes, itching and inflamed eyelids, extreme sensitivity to light, ocular tension, pain in the pupils, rough and dry skin, dry hair (dandruff) lack of appetite, low weight, sterility, stunted growth, malformation of the bones, poor sense of smell, problems of the nervous system, degeneration of the kidneys and other glands, exhaustion and spots.

**Foods that contain vitamin A:** flower pollen, amaranth, bananas, plums, and raspberries. Yellow fruit rich in carotene: apricots, mangoes, cantaloupes, grapes, papaya, pineapple, oranges, and tangerines. Green vegetables: alfalfa, avocado, Romaine lettuce, watercress, celery, cucumber, asparagus and Mexican squash, sweet potatoes and fresh broad beans. Yellow-pigment vegetables: carrots, beetroot, red cabbage, chambray onions, dandelion leaves, turnip leaves and mustard leaves. Red fruit and vegetables: watermelon and red tomatoes. Egg yolk, whole milk, and butter. Dry chile: pasilla, guajillo and morita. Seaweed (nori).

**Herbs that contain vitamin A:** alfalfa, garlic, parsley, red pepper, piquín chili, comfrey, chamomile, dandelion, echinacea, dong quai, fenugreek, eyebright, fennel, ginger, black cohosh, ginseng, burdock, golden rod, marshmallow, sage, rosemary, sarsaparilla, red clover and yarrow.

# B Complex

B complex vitamins are a group of vitamins that depend bio-chemically on each other, so they should be consumed together to provide all the nutritional requirements that the organism needs. The correct balance is seven to eight vitamins B. The organism needs them for the metabolic process that controls all physical and mental energy; if any vitamin is missing, metabolism fails. It is considered as an anti-stress vitamin essential for people who smoke, drink alcohol and coffee.

All vitamin B are eliminated when food is over-processed, so the organism must replace them from its reserves. The body does not store vitamin B very well. Processed food, candies, antibiotics, yeast, alcohol, and tobacco cause serious deficiencies in vitamin B.

Vitamin B helps in cases of nervousness, changes of mood, irritability, depression, anxiety attacks, insomnia, tiredness, fatigue, dizziness, nausea, headache, trembling, tension, hypoglycemia, loss of hair, low level of immunity system, skin problems, acne, problems of the digestive system and sexual impotence, in addition to which it reduces cholesterol, increases appetite, increases energy and keeps the liver healthy. It prevents beriberi, pellagra, athlete's foot, softening of the gums, dry and burning eyes and some types of anemia. Deficiency in complex B vitamins, particularly niacin, may cause dementia, dermatitis and diarrhea.

## Vitamin B-1 (Thiamin)

This vitamin is essential for growth and keeping a health appetite, and also aids digestion and keeps the nerves healthy. This vitamin has anti-neuritis and anti-beriberi properties. The small intestine absorbs it quickly. The circulatory system transports it to the heart, liver and kidneys where, combined with some amino acids (proteins) and manganese, it produces active enzymes.

The presence of vitamin B-1, or thiamine, is important for the use of sugars and carbohydrates, and therefore it helps to digest starch and nourish the nervous system. B-1 hyper-vitaminosis is antagonistic of vitamin B-2, so it is recommendable to consume it from a natural source, such as yeast.

**Deficiency is caused by:** consuming too much cooked food, alcohol, caffeine, sulfa medicines, sugar, white flour and processed food. Daily dose: 1.5 mg.

**Health a benefits:** metabolism of carbohydrates and proteins; it stabilizes the appetite, improves mental attitude, the muscular tone of the stomach, intestine and heart, balances the number of red blood cells and eases your mood and the nervous system. It is useful in cases of arthritis, gout, rheumatism, and nervous disorders in general.

**Problems caused by deficiency:** neuralgia, headache, difficulty in breathing, numb hands and feet, general weakness, irregular heart function, constipation, loss of appetite, weight and memory and ulcers in the cornea.

**Foods that contain this vitamin:** yeast, whole wheat, wheat bran (thiamine is found in the husk of nearly all cereals), wheat germ, whole grain and whole cereal, whole grain rice, soy beans, nuts, seeds, eggs, dairy products, molasses, green-leafed vegetables, beetroot, carrots, cabbage, celery, radishes, red tomatoes, onions, lettuce, cucumber, grapes, papaya, pineapple and cantaloupe.

**Herbs that contain this vitamin:** alfalfa, garlic, cascara sagrada, piquín chile, red pepper, dandelion, fenugreek, ginger, eyebright, licorice, golden rod, marshmallow, great mullein, black cohosh, red clover, burdock and chickweed.

## Vitamin B-2 (Riboflavin)

This vitamin is essential for growth, and helps respiration of the tissues.

Vitamin B-2, Riboflavin or lactoflavin, together with phosphates, forms part of the yellow element of respiration in general. It should be provided regularly as part of your diet, as only small quantities are stored. It is absorbed in the small intestine. Blood transports it to all the body's tissues, the liver and the kidneys. It is not destroyed by heat, oxidation or ultraviolet light. When the body feels tense the need for vitamin B-2 increases, as well as when you are taking drugs, sulfa medicine, alcohol, estrogen and sugar. A large dose does not do any harm.

**Health benefits:** growth and reproduction, cellular respiration and is useful for problems in development and cutaneous alteration of the mucus, nails, hair and the cornea; it alleviates sores on the mouth, lips and tongue; helps to absorb iron and prevents cancer; aids the absorption of oxygen in the blood and the production of red blood cells; relieves headaches. A high dose reduces the frequency of migraine.

**Problems caused by deficiency:** muscular cramp, conjunctivitis, digestive problems, laziness, anemia, tiredness, baldness, dryness on the face, nose and earlobes, sensitivity to light, depression, dizziness, hysteria hypochondria, vaginal itching, difficulty or inability to urinate, headache, stomach afflictions, damage to the skin and mucus, atrophy of the nails, facial dermatitis, and damage to the mucus of the corners of the mouth.

**Food that contains vitamin B-2:** yeast, wheat germ (in the germ of all cereals), grain (whole), whole cereals, rice, legumes, including avocado, green-leafed vegetables, milk, cheese, yoghurt, dairy products, egg yolk, walnuts, almonds, sunflower seed, molasses, seaweed, papaya, grapes and all food that contains vitamin B-1.

**Herbs that contain vitamin B-2:** alfalfa, parsley, dandelion, ginger, fenugreek, eyebright, golden rod, marshmallow, licorice, cascara sagrada, great mullein, black cohosh, red pepper, piquín chili, chickweed and red clover.

## Vitamin B-3 (Niacin)

Take 20 mg a day. High quantities help to reduce the level of cholesterol (under medical supervision). It is involved in some energy production processes. It is called the vitamin of happiness or joy, and is one of the most important of the B complex group. It is also called vitamin PP or PP factor (prevents and cures pellagra, mental illness, depression with delirium, violence and death. Its symptoms are: diarrhea, skin wounds and afflictions of the nervous system).

This vitamin plays a part in the transformation and use of food and is essential in cellular metabolism. It is the tool that uses an important enzyme to repair and fix DNA (the cell's genetic material) that is released by rupture. Niacin has protective properties.

Vitamin B-3 is also called nicotinic acid. It is absorbed in the small intestine and is mainly stored in the liver. Metabolism may produce a certain quantity of vitamin B-3 if the tryptophan amino acid (that forms part of the many proteins that we eat in vegetables and whole cereals) is used.

When people with a deficiency of this vitamin consume it, it may cause redness of the skin that lasts for 10-15 minutes. Another form of vitamin B-3 is niacin amide or nicotine amide that does not cause reddening of the skin like niacin does. It is recommendable to take an equal quantity of niacin than inositol with meals or with vitamin B complex. Sulfa medication, sleeping pills, alcohol, estrogens, processed food and sugar destroy this vitamin.

**Health benefits:**  the nervous system, migraine, autism and mental afflictions, the metabolism of proteins, carbohydrates and fats; it improves the function of the digestive system (in some cases of constipation and diarrhea) and the circulatory system; it is needed to synthesize the sexual hormones, and helps give you a healthy skin, corrects gastrointestinal problems in general and reduces cholesterol.

**Problems caused by deficiency:**  apoplexy, depression, hostility, unnecessary worry, lack of sense of humor, changing personality, hyperactivity, lack of memory, headache and backache, digestive problems, halitosis (bad breath), poor functioning of gastric secretion, alterations in growth, reddened and rough skin sensible to sunlight, dementia, dermatitis and diarrhea.

**Food that contains vitamin B-3:**  yeast, whole wheat, wheat germ, wheat bran, whole grain rice, whole cereal, beans, dairy products, sunflower seeds, almonds, oleaginous products, roasted peanuts, avocado, figs, dates, plums, prunes, papaya, grapes, pineapple, cantaloupe, green vegetables, carrot, cauliflower, celery, broad beans, turnip, seaweed, raw spinach and any dark-green vegetables.

**Herbs that contain vitamin B-3:**  alfalfa, parsley, piquín chili, red pepper, eyebright, dandelion, ginger, fenugreek, marshmallow, licorice, great mullein, golden rod, burdock, chickweed and red clover.

## Vitamin B-4 (Adenine)

This vitamin maintains the balance of white blood cells. It is radio-protective, antitoxic and very necessary for the metabolism of alcohol. Along with other vitamins of group B, it helps normal metabolism of lipids, glucose and protides.

**Foods that contain vitamin B-4:**  yeast, germinated wheat, whole grain rice, whole cereal, oleaginous products, dairy products and green-leafed vegetables.

**Herbs that contain vitamin B-4:**  alfalfa, parsley, red pepper, dandelion, ginger, fenugreek, eyebright, licorice and red clover.

## Vitamin B-5 (Pantothenic Acid or Pantenol)

Vitamin B-5, also called FF factor and filter factor, is a growth factor that is found in various types of food. It is present in all living cells and may be produced by beneficial bacteria in the intestines. This vitamin is necessary for the use of cholin and PABA. It seems that vitamin B-5 stimulates the pituitary gland to produce natural cortisone.

**It is destroyed by:** sleeping tablets, sulfa medicines, processed foods (particularly canned food), estrogen, alcohol, caffeine and sugar.

**Health benefits**: reduces stress and the damaging effect of some antibiotics; it helps the metabolism of proteins, fats and carbohydrates; reduces the formation of flatulence and paralysis of the intestine; it provides resistance to infections and develops antibiotics or bodily defenses. Taken with calcium it detains bruxism (grinding the teeth when asleep). It also helps against hypoglycemia, eases sore throat (chronic), aids cellular respiration and protects blood globules. It also helps in dermatitis, pigmentation of the pilose system, growth problems and the nervous system.

**Problems caused by deficiency:** Neuritis, hypoglycemia, hypoadrenia (exhaustion of the suprarenal glands), allergies, hay fever, blood and skin disorders, anemia, baldness, gray hair, aging, kidneys, the thyroid gland, the sexual glands, healthy cells, stomach and duodenal ulcers, headache, stomach ache, cramp and possibly arthritis.

**Food that contains vitamin B-5:** yeast, wheat germ, wheat bran, whole cereals, beans, peanuts, oleaginous products, egg yolk, dairy products, raw vegetables, algae, raw molasses, honey and royal jelly.

**Herbs that contains vitamin B-5:** alfalfa, parsley, red pepper, piquín chili, dandelion, cascara sagrada, ginger, fenugreek, horse tail, eyebright, marshmallow, licorice, great mullein, burdock, black cohosh, chickweed, red clover, and seaweed (focus vesiculosus).

## Vitamin B-6 (Pyridoxine)

This vitamin is essential for the formation of hemoglobin and for growth, and helps to keep the nerves in good condition.

Vitamin B-6 is found in nearly all foods, particularly in honey, yeast and liver. It helps the metabolism of proteins, glucose, fats, and aids in the absorption of vitamin B-12. It helps to regulate the balance between sodium and potassium and balance the organism's liquids. It is needed for the production of red blood cells, hydrochloric acid, antibiotics and is essential for the synthesis and activity of RNA and DNA. Taken during pregnancy it controls dizziness.

**Health benefits**: conversion of tryptophan (an essential amino acid), nervous tension and premenstrual anxiety, eczema, acne, seborrhea, anemia, hemorrhoids and ulcers. It also helps some problems of the heart, reduces cholesterol, sexual disorders in men, kidney stones, Parkinson's disease and certain types of diabetes.

When this vitamin is deficient, the organs affected include the nervous system and the brain. People that need large quantities of pyridoxine include those who take contraceptives, drink alcohol, smoke and need a lot of protein.

**It is destroyed by**: alcohol, estrogen, processed food, canned food and food stored for a long time.

**Problems caused by deficiency:** deficiency of this vitamin affects the nervous system and the brain. People that need large quantities of pyridoxine include those who take contraceptives, drink alcohol, smoke and need a lot of protein. Deficiency also causes depression, nervousness, chilblains, acne, loss of hair, broken skin around the mouth and eyes, insomnia, slow learning, weak muscles, cramp in the legs and arms, increase in urine, general weakness, poor sight, sensitivity to insulin, heart failure, arteriosclerosis, and digestive and skin problems. Attributed to diabetes.

**Foods that contain vitamin B-6:** yeast, whole grain rice, wheat germ, wheat bran, soy beans, bananas, melons, papaya, grapes, pineapple, carrots, avocado, cabbage, green-leafed vegetables, peppers, radishes, celery, carrots, lettuce, beetroot, red tomatoes, cucumber, algae, dairy products, egg yolk, oleaginous products, peanuts and molasses.

**Herbs that contain vitamin B-6:** alfalfa, parsley, red pepper, cayenne, dandelion, ginger, fenugreek, eyebright, chickweed, cascara sagrada, golden rod, marshmallow, licorice, great mullein, red clover and burdock.

# Vitamin B-9 (Folic acid)

Important for producing white and red blood cells.

It is an anti-anemic vitamin *par excellence*. It reinforces the effects of vitamin B-12 as far as red blood cells are concerned. It helps the organism to produce red blood cells, hydrochloric acid and to improve cell reproduction, as well as in the metabolism of proteins and sugars. It is an important element in the production or synthesis of DNA and RNA. Vitamin B-9 is essential for the production of proteins; it supports a group of enzymes that corrects the defects of genetic DNA material. It also indirectly helps the immunity system.

Healthy intestines may produce some folic acid. It is produced by the synthesis of three chemical substances are: para-aminobenzoic acid (PABA), glutamic acid (amino acid) and pteridine.

**It is destroyed by:** overcooking, sodas, tranquilizers, sulfa medicines, aspirin, anti acids, smoking, medication for high pressure, anti-inflammatory medication, anti-convulsive medication, diuretics and medication that reduces cholesterol.

**Health benefits:** prevents gray hair and sores on the mouth, menstruation, problems of gout and arteriosclerosis; it rebuilds the organism and prevents food poisoning, increases appetite and intelligence, prevents complications involving pregnancy and breast feeding and prevents anemia.

**Problems caused by deficiency:** gastro-intestinal problems, gray hair, weakness, confusion, sores, fatigue, mental disturbances, irritability, insomnia, poor memory, isolation, schizophrenia, intestinal problems associated with diarrhea and fatigue, headache, red and smooth tongue, dysplastic cells, and susceptibility to cancer. It prevents congenital defects of the fetus during the first four critical weeks of development.

**Foods that contain vitamin B-9:** yeast, whole wheat, whole barley, beans, whole cereals, egg yolk, peanuts, oleaginous products, green-leafed vegetables such as spinach asparagus, chard, broccoli, Brussels' sprouts, avocado, peas, corn, parsley, beetroot leaves. beet, apricots, cantaloupe, papaya, pineapple and algae.

**Herbs that contain vitamin B-9:** alfalfa, parsley, red pepper, cayenne, cascara sagrada, eyebright, dandelion, fenugreek, ginger, licorice root, great mullein, marshmallow, golden rod, burdock, red clover and seaweed (focus vesiculosus).

## Vitamin B-12 (Cobalamin)

Vitamin B-12 is stored in the organism and prevents and cures anemia. Vitamin B-12 is best combined with calcium. It plays an important role in many metabolic functions and it may also use vitamin D and some amino acids. It contributes to the use of iron and is essential for the production and maturity of red blood cells.

People with vitamin B-12 deficiency develop pernicious anemia (prevented by vitamins B-12 and B-9)

**It is destroyed by:** sunlight, sleeping pills and alcohol.

**Health benefits:** prevents insomnia and nervousness, improves concentration, reduces irritability and skin problems, and increases energy and coordination. Also used for anemia and asthma.

**Problems caused by deficiency:** pernicious anemia, physical and mental damage, palpitations, flatulence, constipation, diarrhea, poor appetite and vomiting, dryness of head skin (dandruff), ringing in the ears and growth problems.

**Foods that contain vitamin B-12 :** yeast, raw wheat germ, sunflower seeds, seaweed, flower pollen, grapes, pineapple, melon, bananas, papaya, carrots, beetroot, cabbage, celery, radishes, red tomatoes, onions, cucumber, lettuce, eggs, dairy products and Roquefort cheese (a natural antibiotic). It is suggested that vegetarians take a vitamin B-12 supplement.

**Herbs that contain vitamin B-12 :** alfalfa, celery, red pepper, cayenne, dandelion, eyebright, dong-quai, ginger, fenugreek, cascara sagrada, Siberian ginseng. licorice, great mullein, marshmallow, golden rod, red clover and seaweed (focus vesiculosus).

## Vitamin B-15 (Pangamic acid)

Stimulates the immunity system.

**Health benefits:**   protects against environmental pollution, protects the liver, helps reduce fatigue, and prolongs the life of cells. Its antagonists are sunlight and water.

**Foods that contain vitamin B-15:** fresh and raw fruit, raw vegetables and whole grain.

**Herbs that contain vitamin B-15:** black nuts.

## Vitamin B-17 (Laetrile)

Laetrile contains natural cyanide.

**Foods that contain vitamin B-17:** apricot and apple pips, peaches, apples, cherries, nectarines and plums.

## Choline

Belongs to the B complex group and it is manufactured by a healthy organism. It is a lecithin compound that goes to the brain to help to its production. Lecithin emulsifies fats and together with inositol it dissolves and utilizes fats and cholesterol.

**It is destroyed by:** processed foods, alcohol, sulfa medication, estrogen and water.

**Health benefits:** relieves cramp caused by circulatory blockage; regulates high blood pressure, improves and recovers loss of memory; it helps the liver by releasing poison (in viral hepatitis) and keeps it healthy; it also helps the functioning of the gallbladder, spleen and thymus, and relieves diabetes, arteriosclerosis, muscular dystrophy.

**Problems caused by deficiency:** liver, high blood pressure, bleeding stomach, ulcers, blocks the tracks of the kidneys and causes hemorrhages, in the nervous system, insomnia, nervous ticks, poor sight, dizziness, buzzing in the ears and problems with growth.

**Foods that contain choline:** alfalfa, cayenne, red pepper, eyebright, dandelion, fenugreek, ginger, licorice, cascara sagrada, great mullein, marshmallow, golden rod, red clover and seaweed (focus vesiculosus).

## Coenzyme Q-10

A powerful natural antioxidant that is vital for the production of energy. If its level decreases your general state of health also decreases. The ideal dose is 50 mg per day.

It is excellent for preventing and delaying aging; it protects the mitochondria; it protects and strengthens the liver, the cardiovascular system and the immunity system. It is essential for the skin and hair and provides a high degree of resistance to tumors.

## Vitamin C (ascorbic acid)

Important for absorbing iron, healing processes, forming defenses and reducing the risk of infections.

Vitamin C is also called the anti scurvy vitamin (scurvy is a serious illness whose symptoms include slimness, muscular, bone, and digestive disorders and frequent hemorrhages).

The body does not produce this vitamin (not even the lysine amino acid). You should take around 150 mg daily to maintain health. Heat and oxygen destroy this vitamin quickly. It is an antioxidant, protects the cells (protects the genetic code) and strengthens the immunity system. It builds collagen, elastin, and the body's connective tissues. It is antitoxic and provides protection against of all types of poisons. It neutralizes mental and physical stress and strengthens the capillary wall. It helps the absorption of iron and glucose and is essential for the proper functioning of the suprarenal glands and the thyroid gland. It specifically helps in gastro-intestinal problems, ensures the integrity of blood vessels and blood circulation. It is also essential for normal development of bones and regulates the nutrition of the entire conjunctive tissue. It is important for synthesizing steroid hormones and for capillary resistance and healing.

If you take a large dose, take it with complex B and calcium. Increase the dose if you live in a polluted city, if you suffer from stress, drink alcohol, smoke, take aspirin (for pain), contraceptives, etc. If you are suffering from emotional tension take 500 mg daily. Vitamin C and collagen strengthen the circulatory system.

**It is destroyed by:** high temperatures (cooking) and exposure of food to air and light (oxidation).

**Health benefits:** Helps diabetes, cancer, eye infections; it prevents cataracts and ulcers, helps the suprarenal glands, relieves gallstones and throat infections (cold), pyorrhea, sterility or impotence; it keeps the protein cells together and prevents wrinkles; improves the flexibility of the joints, controls stress and may be used for treating hepatitis; attacks viral and bacterial infections; helps to keep the mind alert (mental agility), removes polyps in the colon, heals burns and wounds, prevents blood clotting, makes birth easier and more healthy, acts as a natural antibiotic, combats fatigue, and protects smokers. It is the best possible relief for stress.

**Problems caused by deficiency:** general weakness of the teeth and bones, anemia, and problems of the digestive-intestinal system; inflammation and pain in joints, bleeding gums, nasal hemorrhages, bruising, irritability, rheum, tiredness, and high levels of cholesterol. Dr. Rath says that vitamin C, lysine and proline are an excellent for AIDS and that lysine prevents the spreading of cancer.

**Foods that contain vitamin C:** all fresh fruit, particularly citric fruits such as oranges, limes, mandarins, grapefruit, haw fruit, apples, guavas, kiwi fruit, strawberries, red currants, papaya, pineapple, Chinese melon and honeydew melon, mangoes, cherimoya, custard apple, quinces, watermelon, grapes, litchi, sapodilla, and black and white raisins; all fresh vegetables: parsley, peas, yucca, red and green pepper, small tomatoes, red tomatoes, broccoli, cabbage, carrots, beetroot, celery, cucumber, onions, radishes, lettuce, potatoes, turnip leaf, lotus root and sweet potatoes; green vegetables, flower pollen, rose petals, nori seaweed and cow's milk.

**Herbs that contain vitamin C:** alfalfa, garlic, parsley, thyme, ginger, mint, common comfrey, dandelion, eyebright, red pepper, cayenne, echinacea, barberry, fennel, golden rod, burdock, yarrow, red clover, mint, and seaweed (focus vesiculosus).

## Vitamin D (Calciferol)

Called the anti-rachitic, solar and nerves vitamin. Its most important role is facilitating the absorption of calcium in the intestine and incorporating calcium salts into the bones and teeth.

In the organism, vitamin D is transformed by the pro-vitamin ergosterol (found in vegetables) and the cholesterol under the skin, by means of ultraviolet rays (gradual exposure to sun in the morning is recommended) and it is distributed throughout the entire body by the circulatory system. The organism stores this vitamin, particularly in the liver and in the suprarenal capsules in order to face winter. It helps the assimilation of calcium, phosphorous, and other minerals needed for maintaining the joints and nervous system. It is important for normal development of teeth and bones, particularly during childhood, adolescence and pregnancy. People who live in polluted areas should supervise their intake of vitamin D which produces melanin that is a regulator. It is recommended that only natural (organic) vitamins be taken. Synthetic vitamin D in excess has a toxic effect.

**Health benefits:** heals fractures, prevents tooth decay and keeps the teeth strong and the skin healthy. Helps assimilate vitamin A, and absorb calcium and phosphorous.

**Problems caused by deficiency:** rickets in children, deformity of the bones (softening of the bones and osteoporosis), tooth decay, muscular cramp, weak muscles, irritation of the joints, weak nervous system, gas, constipation, diarrhea, nervous disorders, pellagra (depressive mental illness), dementia, insomnia, scaly and rough skin, dermatitis, and breaking of the calcium phosphate balance in adults who do not receive enough sunlight. Causes calcium deficiency and is associated with cardiac disease, and cancer of the colon and the prostate gland.

**Foods that contain vitamin D:** seaweed, sprouts, sunflower seeds, mushrooms, papaya, flower pollen, egg yolk, milk, and butter.

**Herbs that contain vitamin D:** alfalfa, fenugreek, great mullein, eyebright and sarsaparilla.

# Vitamin E (Tocopherol)

A powerful antioxidant; active in reproductive functions and preserves skin tissue.

Tocopherol is from the Greek *tokos* = "child birth" or "descendants", and *pherin* = "produce".

It is called the fertility of reproduction vitamin and it naturally dilutes the blood (without causing hemorrhages). Tocopherol also means "the ability to create youth". Vitamin E is useful for everything. On its own, it is used as an anti-aging treatment because it protects oxidation of the cells. The organism stores it for a short time and removes any excess through feces. It is recommendable to take 50 mg a day. It is antioxidant and "prevents auto-oxidation of very unsaturated fatty acids when they are exposed to molecular oxygen". Manganese must be present so that vitamin E has an effect on the organism.

It reduces the level of cholesterol if taken with vitamin A. Vitamins E and C taken with selenium increases its power as a cellular antioxidant, protecting the cells against premature aging and hardening of the tissues caused by oxidation; vitamins E, C and A protect the eyes; vitamins E and K help good coagulation; vitamin E protects the cellular membrane against attack by of super-oxides and free radicals (the nervous system is particularly vulnerable to this attack) and maintains the strength of the immunity system. It is also involved in the synthesis of proteins and aids spermatogenesis.

Vitamin E sometimes works slowly and gradually, because the body has its own rhythm or adjusts to the improvement. Under some conditions it works very quickly. It seems that a rheumatic heart responds better to a small dose, as does high blood pressure.

**It is destroyed by**: cooking, high or very low temperature, mineral oils, inorganic iron, chlorine, processes and fried food.

**Health benefits:** cells surviving with less oxygen; expanding and dilating blood vessels; improves blood circulation; strengthens the activity of vitamin A and invigorates and strengthens muscles; it relieves muscular dystrophy (taken in high doses); it helps for all menstrual problems, prevents fibrosis in the breasts, prevents wrinkles, removes dark blotches on the skin caused by liver problems, heals wounds, alleviates cardiac problems and protects the lungs against contamination, cramp, tiredness, Parkinson's disease, inflammation of the pancreas, diabetes, helps the kidneys and the liver. It prevents cancer, abortion, arteriosclerosis and myocardium infarction. It is anti-inflammatory, anti-dementia, and helps to maintain the spirit of physical and mental youth. It generally protects all cells, particularly the nerve cells, protects the lung tissues and provides protection against tumors. It may reduce prostate cancer by up to 50%.

**Problems caused by deficiency:** anemia (destruction of red blood cells), all problems related to the reproductive system: lack of sexual interest, sterility, abortion, etc.; weakness or muscular degeneration, skin problems, loss of hair, cardiac problems, poor coagulation, hemorrhages, itching and numbness in the toes and hands, loss of coordination and visual sensitivity, cataracts and pulmonary emphysema.

**Foods that contain vitamin E:** "extra virgin" vegetable oils (cold pressed), wheat germ oil, soy oil, particularly Omega 3 oils, whole wheat, wheat germ, whole cereals, grain, seaweed, papaya, mangoes, apples, sweet potatoes, bean sprouts, green-leafed vegetables, spinach, lettuce, Brussels sprouts, broccoli, avocado, eggs, molasses, oleaginous products and flower pollen.

**Herbs that contain vitamin E:** alfalfa, dandelion, echinacea, dong-quai, eyebright, common comfrey, golden rod, Siberian ginseng, licorice, yarrow, burdock, and seaweed (focus vesiculosus).

## Vitamin F (linoleic acid)

Vitamin F comprises unsaturated fatty acids. The organism does not make them so they must be taken in the form of pressed oils (cold-extracted), corn oil, sunflower or soy oil.

Moderate consumption helps weight loss; excess consumption increases weight. It is best taken with meals. One of its most important functions is to support the glandular function, mainly the thyroid gland and suprarenal glands.

**It is destroyed by:** saturated fats, oxygen, heat and fried food.

**Health benefits:** protects the skin and treats acne and eczema. It is healthy for the nervous system, mucus, cells and hair. It regulates blood coagulation, protects the damaging effects of X-rays and combats afflictions of the heart.

**Problems caused by deficiency:** acne, eczema, dry skin and hair, edemas (bruising), varicose veins, low weight, little beneficial bacteria in the intestine, diarrhea, absence of sexual desire, ovulation and spermatogenesis deficiency, growth problems, gallstones and accumulation of cholesterol.

**Foods that contain vitamin F :** cotton seed oil, soy oil, corn oil, sunflower oil and peanut oil. All seeds, peanuts, nuts (except Brazil nuts), almonds, and strawberries, avocado and wheat germ.

**Herb that contains vitamin F:** yarrow.

## Vitamin H-1 (Biotin)

Vitamin H belongs to the complex B group. It exists in all living tissues in small quantities. It may be synthesized by beneficial intestine bacteria. It is needed for the metabolism of proteins, fats, (and unsaturated fatty acids) and vitamin F. It plays a role in growth phenomena. Lack of this vitamin may cause atrophy of muscular tissue, testicular degeneration and seborrheic dermatitis in children. Raw eggs white contain avidine that inhibit the absorption of biotin. Men who loose the hair, people who take sulfa medication (antibiotics), drink alcohol, eat processed food and take estrogen should take extra vitamin H, as should women who are breast feeding, even though breast milk contains biotin. If the intestinal flora is healthy and abundant it may synthesize this vitamin.

**Health benefits:** helps baldness, prevents gray hair and aids normal growth; also contributes to the good health of the bone medulla, the nervous system, skin, the sebaceous glands, the mind and the hair. It helps the sexual glands to function properly, decreases muscular discomfort and combats depression and somnolence.

**Problems caused by deficiency:** tiredness, loss of energy, mental and emotional depression, insomnia, loss of hair, rapid propagation of cancer, lack of appetite, vomiting, nausea, muscular pain and pain around the area of the heart.

**Foods that contain vitamin H-1 :** yeast, seaweed, whole cereal, (rice, wheat, oats), wheat germ, beans, soy beans, peanuts, oleaginous products, dairy products, egg yolk and papaya.

**Herbs that contain vitamin H-1 :** alfalfa, red pepper, cayenne, licorice, cascara sagrada, great mullein, red clover, marshmallow, and seaweed (focus vesiculosus).

## Vitamin I (Inositol)

Part of the B complex group. Inositol and choline form lecithin. In a healthy body, there is more inositol than any other vitamin, except for vitamin B-3 (niacin). It is found in abundance in the heart muscle and in the brain, where there are very high concentrations. Women after menopause and people who drink alcohol, caffeine, take sulfa medicine, eat processed food and take estrogen should consume extra quantities of inositol. Take inositol with vitamin E for treating the nervous system.

**Health benefits:** prevents baldness, circulatory problems, arteriosclerosis, diabetes, standardizes the eyes (strabismus, etc), gallbladder, metabolizes and distributes fats, reduces levels of cholesterol, mental retardation, paralysis of the brain, multiple dystrophy; stimulates cerebral activity, protects the heart, kidneys and liver and corrects the proper functioning of the heart muscle.

**Problems caused by deficiency:** eczema (various diseases of the skin), loss of hair, abnormalities in the eyes, constipation and high levels of cholesterol.

**Foods that contain vitamin I:** yeast, lecithin, egg yolk, untreated milk, yoghurt, vegetables and soy beans; whole cereals: rice, wheat, oats, etc., wheat germ, whole meal bread, beans, seaweed, oleaginous products, peanuts, cabbage, cantaloupe, papaya, raisins, milk and molasses.

**Herbs that contain vitamin I:** alfalfa, cayenne, red pepper, eyebright, dandelion, ginger, cascara sagrada, golden rod, great mullein, licorice, marshmallow, red clover and seaweed (focus vesiculosus).

## Vitamin K (Menadine)

This is a coagulating vitamin produced by beneficial intestinal bacteria (the main source) in healthy people. It helps the liver to produce prothrombin that, together with vitamin K, turns into thrombin, a coagulating agent. It needs biliary secretion to be used and it stimulates considerably the normal function of the liver.

**Health benefits:** normal blood coagulation reduces hemorrhages and controls excessive menstruation.

**Problems caused by deficiency:** internal hemorrhaging in the nose and mouth, diarrhea, colitis, poor coagulation of the blood, deficient absorption of nutrients, and varicose veins.

**Foods that contain vitamin K:** corn, wheat germ, beans, cow's milk, yoghurt, all dairy products, egg yolk, seaweed, spiruline seaweed, soy oil, green-leafed vegetables, spinach, carrots, cabbage, cauliflower, Brussels' sprouts, broccoli, potatoes, red tomatoes, peas, strawberries, papaya and bee's honey (produced by bees extracted from clover fields).

**Herbs that contain vitamin K:** alfalfa, gotu-kola and yarrow.

## Vitamin P (Bioflavonoids)

The bioflavonoid complex is made up of citrine, rutin and hesperidin.

It works together with vitamin C to keep the cells' connective tissue (collagen) healthy, and helps the capillary vessels to control their small orifice to just allow nutrients through, at the same time blocking viruses or waste (that may cause illness) or red blood cells (that may cause hemorrhages). It is destroyed or inhibited by light, high temperature (cooking) water, cigarettes and air.

**Health benefits:** strengthens the capillary walls, regulates coagulation (protects against excess), treats asthma, ulcers, edemas (a natural diuretic) and dizziness caused by problems in the inner ear. It also cures and prevents bleeding gums and prevents degeneration of the arteries.

**Problems caused by deficiency:** diabetes, hemorrhoids, bruising and easy bleeding of the nose and gums, etc. excessive menstrual bleeding, habitual and spontaneous threat of abortion, skin problems, edema and rhinitis.

**Food that contains vitamin P:** the pulp and peel of all fruit and vegetables and the white of the peel of citric fruits (limes, oranges and grapefruits); dry and fresh plums, cherries, apricots, all types of berries, melon, buckwheat, red tomatoes, broccoli, spinach and paprika.

**Herbs that contain vitamin P:** cayenne, red pepper, dandelion, red clover and burdock.

## Vitamin T

This vitamin increases the number of platelets that play an important role in coagulation of the blood, as vitamin K does.

**Foods that contain vitamin T :** egg yolk and some oils, such as sesame seed oil.

## Vitamin  U

This is a little-known vitamin, but it is important for treating and curing gastric, septic and duodenal ulcers. It is destroyed by cooking (heat).

**Foods that contain vitamin U:** raw cabbage, cabbage juice, raw celery, celery juice, raw green vegetables, untreated milk and egg yolk (raw).

**Herbs that contain vitamin U:** alfalfa.

## PABA  (Para-Amino Benzoic Acid)

This vitamin is part of the complex B group. PABA is produced in the intestines under suitable conditions and it helps in producing folic acid (vitamin B-9) in the intestines. It is also one of the basic parts of folic acid. PABA and folic acid restore the natural color of hair.

**It is destroyed by:** sulfa medication (may produce PABA deficiency and deficiency of pantothenic and folic acid), estrogen, processed food, alcohol and water.

**Health benefits:** metabolizes protein, keeps the intestine healthy, assimilates pantothenic acid (vitamin B-5), protects the skin from the sun, delays aging, reduces pain caused by burns and may be used to treat vitiligo and help conception in women.

**Problems caused by deficiency:** eczema (various skin diseases), racked nerves, irritability, depression, hallucinations, tiredness and poor digestion.

**Foods that contain PABA:** yeast, whole grain, whole grain rice, wheat germ, wheat bran, seaweed, papaya, dairy products, such as yoghurt, and eggs and molasses.

**Herbs that contain PABA:** alfalfa, red pepper, cayenne, eyebright, dandelion, ginger, golden rod, fenugreek, cascara sagrada, horse tail, licorice, red clover, great mullein, marshmallow, burdock and seaweed (focus vesiculosus).

# A Glance At Minerals

All forms of life directly or indirectly
depend on plants to feed themselves

Minerals are vital in the basic process of life. They play a major role in activating several vitamins, as well as in cellular nutrition, construction and maintenance of the structural system, metabolism, digestion, assimilation of food and chemical composition of all tissues.

Organic minerals are produced by nature's processes; inorganic minerals are part of the earth itself. They are diminutive crystals of mineral salts that commence their transformation into organic minerals through microbes that live in the soil, a process that continues when plants absorb them.

There is an abundance of minerals (organic minerals) in the plant kingdom that are similar to our body. We should provide our body fresh minerals due to its constant change. Refined food "steals" essential minerals from the organism that leads to many afflictions. Deficiency could bring about bad diet and problems in absorption.

Minerals are classified as macro-minerals and oligoelements. Macro minerals are those that we must consume daily in quantities of 2 to 3 grams and include sulfur, chloride, calcium, phosphorous, magnesium, phosphorous and sodium. Oligoelements are those that we should consume in on smaller quantities, less than 45 mg per kilo of weight. These minerals include boride, copper, cobalt, chrome, tin, strontium, fluorine, iron, molybdenum, manganese, nickel, lead, silica, selenium, vanadium, iodine and zinc.

## Trace minerals

Trace minerals are obtained from the depth of the soil where roots reach a depth of 9 to 30 meters. Trace minerals, or oligoelements, are found in smaller quantities in the organism (it has not been established if they are essential for life). Some of these include bromide, vanadium, nickel and strontium.

**Herbs that contain trace minerals:** alfalfa, sorrel, dandelion, horse tail, cascara sagrada, hawthorn, burdock, leather weed, eyebright, thyme, parsley, sage, valerian, *castella tortuosa*, peppermint, sarsaparilla, and red clover.

## Chelated minerals

The organism dissolves minerals and a protein molecule (hydrolyzed or amino acids), and wraps them, an essential process for the blood flow to accept the mineral.
Sometimes the organism cannot dissolve inorganic hard minerals due to weak or poor digestion. If minerals are taken already chelated, the organism uses them safely.

## Sulfur

Organic sulfur is indispensable for all the basic metabolic functions of the body (inorganic sulfur may cause negative effects). It is important for the formation of active compounds of the nervous system, the brain and the tissues. It is also a part of cartilage and tendons. It purifies and activates the organism. Sulfur is found in an organic combination with albumin and it is for favorable the metabolism of certain reduction and oxidation phenomena. We obtain it from food high in protein. The daily intake of sulfur should be between 1 and 2 grams.

**Helps to:** produce antibodies, metabolize carbohydrates, remove waste (contaminants), produce collagen, keep the skin healthy, the nails strong, and hair shiny, develop and repair tissues and maintain the oxygen balance.

**Problems caused by deficiency:** on the skin: low resistance to the secondary effects of chemical products (medicine) and poison; may cause problems similar to those caused by lack of protein or sulfuric amino acids.

**Foods that contain sulfur:** beans, soy beans, lentils, germinated wheat, oleaginous products, peanuts, hazelnuts, chestnut, eggs, beet, Brussels' sprouts, cabbage, cauliflower, onions, carrots, asparagus, mustard leaves and seaweed.

**Herbs that contain sulfur:** alfalfa, garlic, burdock, cayenne, dandelion, common comfrey, parsley, time, fennel, echinacea, great mullein, sarsaparilla, *castella tortuosa,* lobelia, peppermint, and seaweed (focus vesiculosus).

## Boron

A trace mineral that revitalizes the memory and that is indispensable for activating the hormones that regulate the formation of bone mass. Boron deficiency affects the skeleton and the brain and the metabolism of calcium and magnesium.

**Foods that contain boron:** dry fruit, peanuts, raisins, grapes, and vegetables.

## Calcium

A mineral that is found in our bodies in great quantity, forming part of the skeleton (bones), teeth and soft tissues (90-98% is found in bones and teeth). Bones are a complex, dynamic structure through which minerals, particularly calcium, enter and leave fibrous cells. A daily health dose should be between 500 mg and 800 mg. There should be sufficient vitamin D in the organism to assimilate calcium. Physical exercise maintains levels of calcium. Calcium and magnesium work together for correct cardiovascular functioning. Calcium helps in the functions of vitamin C and plays a role in the process of digestion and assimilation of food. Small quantities of calcium are lost in the urine because it helps to remove waste material.

Old people suffering from emotional stress, people suffering from hypoglycemia, children, pregnant women and women going through menopause should increase their consumption of calcium. It may also be taken for backache, aching muscles, leg ache, growth, arthritis, birth, and for menstrual and muscular cramp. A higher dose alleviates some symptoms of old age. Take exercise (skipping). It is needed to keep up your muscular strength, maintain the function of the nervous system, and keep blood pressure normal and mainly to form vitamin D. Sunbathe.

**The functions of calcium are:** building and maintaining the bone structure, raising the organic tone and the organic process, playing a vital role in the transmission of nerve impulses, heart beat, blood coagulation, muscular contraction, and maintaining the balance of potassium and sodium. It also activates some of the hormones that are needed for metabolism; it counteracts acids, cures wounds, provides vitality and resistance and is a natural tranquilizer.

**Calcium is destroyed by:** oxalic acid and excess fat.

**Helps to:** reduce insomnia, alleviate the nervous system, migraine and rickets, as well as to reduce triglycerides, cholesterol and birth pain; it metabolizes iron; it is useful for skin problems; it reduces muscular tension, cramp, numbness in the extremities, pain in the joints, arthritis and osteoporosis, tension in the neck, bruxism (grinding teeth), back pain, arrhythmia, hypertension, conjunctivitis and cataracts. It prevents cancer of the colon and heart attack. It reduces toxicity caused by lead.

**Problems caused by deficiency:** rickets, muscular weakness, convulsions, multiple sclerosis, insomnia, tooth decay, inflamed gums, cataracts, pain in the joints and in the lower part of the back, curving of the shoulders, osteoporosis (during menopause, because the production of estrogens related to the formation of bones reduces), vitamin D deficiency, causes calcium deficiency and cardiovascular diseases. It helps to reduce tension, cholesterol and the risk of cancer of the colon.

**Foods that contain calcium:** vegetables, beans, tofu (soy cheese ), dairy products, raw egg yolk, egg shell, bran, whole wheat bread, sunflower seeds, walnuts, peanuts, sesame seeds, almonds, prunes, grapes, dates, dried fruit, raspberries, papaya, figs, dark green-leafed vegetables, cabbage, onions, spinach, broccoli, lettuce, asparagus, root vegetables (potato, sweet potato) and seaweed. Orange juice contains calcium and also fixes calcium.

**Herbs that contain calcium:** alfalfa, garlic, common comfrey, cayenne, dandelion, ginger, chamomile, Siberian ginseng, aloe, cascara sagrada, golden rod, marshmallow, sage, parsley, fennel, rosemary and red clover.

## Copper

Copper is a trace mineral or oligoelement that forms part of the enzymes that play a role in digestion. It is an important auxiliary mineral in absorbing iron and synthesizing hemoglobin; it also helps in metabolizing proteins and ascorbic acid. The organism better assimilates copper when it is consumed with small quantities of vitamin C throughout the day. It is obtained from foods such as whole grain, vegetables, oleaginous products, raisins, cherries and your daily intake is just 2 mg. Supervise levels of zinc and copper in the body as excess reduces the levels of zinc.

**Helps:** the nervous system and the liver, to keep coronary arteries strong; it also increases energy, prevents gray hair, makes bones healthy, helps normal growth and calms the nerves. Helps protect the nerves Melina.

**Problems caused by deficiency:** may cause anemia and some alterations in the bones.

**Foods that contain copper:** whole grain (cereals and legumes), dry peas, beans, eggs, almonds, oleaginous products, green-leafed or liquid chlorophyll vegetables, beet, carrots, vegetable broth, prunes, molasses, oranges, cherries, apples, pears, grapes, pineapple and seaweed.

**Herbs that contain copper:** garlic, horse tail, dandelion, red clover, yarrow, common comfrey, echinacea, chickweed, golden rod, eyebright, valerian, peppermint, sarsaparilla and lobelia.

# Cobalt

This mineral is part of vitamin B-12 (cobalamin). The liver stores a little. Cobalamin is essential for the correct production of red blood vessels and plays a major role in the proper functioning of cells. Iron, calcium, and vitamin B-6 support the function of cobalamin.

**It is destroyed by:** alcohol, sleeping pills, sunlight, estrogen and water.

**Helps:** mental agility; metabolizes folic acid, essential fats and proteins; increases energy, digestion of carbohydrates, and helps normal growth.

**Problems caused by deficiency:** pernicious anemia, nervous weakness, palpitations, loss of mental agility, tiredness, diarrhea, insecurity when walking and paralysis.

**Foods that contain cobalt:** yoghurt, Cheddar and Swiss cheese, eggs and seaweed.

**Herbs that contain cobalt:** horse tail, dandelion, red clover, parsley, lobelia, and seaweed (focus vesiculosus).

# Chloride

Chloride is of great help to the digestive system and secretions, because it eliminates waste and cleans, disinfects, purifies and refreshes the organism. It is important for the acid/alkaline balance in forming gastric juice. Chloride plays an active part in forming bones, cartilage and teeth. Your daily intake should be around 15 grams. It is very important for vegetarian diets.

**Problems caused by deficiency:** may cause loss of appetite, muscular cramp and mental apathy.

**Food that contains chloride:** dairy products, cow's milk, goat's milk, eggs, sea salt, seaweed, radish, beetroot, celery, spinach, lettuce, string beans, coconuts, almonds, oleaginous products, hazelnuts, dates, honey and bananas.

# Chrome

A trace mineral or oligoelement. It is only found in small quantities in the organism and only a small quantity of organic chrome is needed. It is very important in aiding metabolism of glucose, as a catalyst of the activity of insulin and in producing energy. It is of great help in preventing hypoglycemia and diabetes and for people who are already suffering from this condition. People suffering from diabetes, old people and pregnant women should consume a large quantity of chrome.

**Destroyed by:** junk food, and refined foods, such as flour, and sugar.

**Problems caused by deficiency:** may be a cause of diabetes because it can decrease the capacity to metabolize glucose and harden the arteries.

**Helps to:** maintain the level of insulin, transport glucose to the cells, metabolize carbohydrates, prevent the formation of cholesterol in the liver, reduce cholesterol, and triglycerides.

**Foods that contain chrome:** yeast, dairy products, whole grain, corn, corn oil, unpeeled potatoes, mushrooms, raw and fresh vegetables, and seaweed.

**Herbs that contain chrome:** licorice and seaweed (focus vesiculosus).

# Fluorine

An essential mineral found in the organism in small quantities, mainly in the bones and teeth (enamel) in the form of fluorides that strengthen the teeth and reduce tooth decay. It acts on the metabolism of calcium, helps to prevent tooth decay and supports consolidation of fractures.

Excess may damage the kidneys, liver, heart, central nervous system, and affect the metabolism of vitamins. Exercise caution with aluminum and fluoride salts.

**Helps to:** weld bones, strengthen tendons, provide resistance against diseases, and make the body more attractive.

**Problems caused by deficiency:** predisposition to tooth decay.

**Food that contains fluorine:** soy beans, whole grain rice, corn, wheat germ, oats, seaweed, grenetine, sunflower seeds, raw egg yolk, cheese, apples, grapefruit, potatoes, cauliflower, cabbage, spinach, red tomatoes, watercress, lettuce, onions and drinking water.

**Herbs that contain fluorine:** alfalfa, hops, black nuts and seaweed (focus vesiculosus).

# Phosphorous

Phosphorous is a mineral that is easily obtained from food, therefore it is abundant throughout our entire organism. A high quantity is found in the teeth and bones and the rest in liquids and cells in the form of adenosine tri-phosphate, which controls the delivery of energy to the organism, increased by magnesium. The acid-alkaline balance is important. It is essential for the nervous system to function correctly, particularly the brain, and for assimilating vitamin B-3 (Niacin). Calcium and vitamin D are essential for the normal function of phosphorous. Excessive consumption of phosphorous may cause loss of calcium through the urine.

**Destroyed by:** consuming too much iron, aluminum and magnesium.

**Helps to:** provide energy, promote cellular metabolism, and produce hormones and lecithin; assimilates proteins, carbohydrates and fats, transform food into energy, and fluids of the body. It also plays an active role in the function of the kidneys, the metabolism of sugar, preserving bone cells and teeth (together with zinc).

**Problems caused by deficiency:** demineralization of the bones, loss of calcium, arthritis, demineralization of teeth and gums, pyorrhea, low weight or overweight, poor growth of bones and weakness.

**Foods that contain phosphorous:** whole grain and cereal, vegetables, eggs, dairy products, all seeds, oleaginous products, raw vegetables, papaya, raspberries and dried fruit.

**Herbs that contain phosphorous:** alfalfa, garlic, barberry, cayenne, black nuts, dandelion, ginger, common comfrey, hawthorn, rosemary, sage, parsley, and seaweed (focus vesiculosus).

# Iron

This is the most important mineral for the production of red blood cells in the blood. The blood transports oxygen to cells and extracts carbon dioxide from them. Keeps energy levels high when receiving sufficient oxygen through hemoglobin. Iron is stored in the liver. Enzymes also contain iron to play their part in the role of muscular functions. Iron is needed to absorb vitamin B.

Vitamin C is needed, along with calcium, cobalt and copper, for the proper assimilation of iron, so that it may carry out its function. Sufficient iron and calcium should be consumed, particularly by women who are the most susceptible to this deficiency (due to menstruation and pregnancy), and older people, as their absorption is worse. People who grow quickly need more iron. It is recommendable to consume only organic iron.

**Destroyed by:** the tonic acid of coffee, and black tea, and phosphates in the form of additives (conserving elements).

**Helps to:** stimulate vitality, provide energy and motivation to win, prevent anemia, provide resistance to tension and illnesses, and provide a good skin tone.

**Problems caused by deficiency:** the most common nutritional deficiency is anemia (the end result of chronic iron deficiency, whose symptoms include diarrhea, insufficient hydrochloric acid in the stomach, diseases of the intestinal tract, acute inflammation of the stomach with wear of its lining – atrophic gastritis-), diarrhea, constipation, flatulence, lack of appetite, nausea when finishing meals, headache, dizziness, general weakness, abnormal tiredness, respiratory problems, depression, nervousness, palpitations, skin and nail problems, lack of concentration, problems of the skin, reduced capacity to fight infections, may cause deficiency, loss of blood due to excessive menstrual hemorrhaging, bleeding ulcers and hemorrhoids.

**Food that contains iron:** yeast, beans, lentils, whole cereals, whole wheat, wheat germ, oats, oleaginous products, sunflower seeds, egg yolk, Gruyere cheese, grapes, raspberries, papaya, dry peaches, apricots, dates, prunes, raisins, and dry fruit. All dark green-leafed vegetables: spinach, broccoli, potato peel, seaweed and brown sugar in a cone. Orange juice increases the absorption of iron.

**Herbs that contain iron:** alfalfa, garlic, chamomile, aloe, cayenne, horse tail, dandelion, fenugreek, common comfrey, eyebright, ginger, echinacea, chickweed, golden rod, parsley, great mullein, Siberian ginseng, marshmallow, red clover, sarsaparilla, yarrow, rosemary, Pau d'arco, lobelia, and hawthorn.

## Magnesium

A mineral that has a calming effect; it is important for metabolizing calcium, phosphorous, potassium, sodium and vitamin C, and for activating enzymatic reactions and synthesis of proteins. Vitamin B-6 (pyridoxine) should be taken with magnesium. Excess magnesium may cause problems for people who have a phosphorous-calcium imbalance.

**Destroyed by:** refined sugar and flour, processed food, alcohol, too much protein, and diuretics.

**Helps:** the nervous system and the digestive system to carry out their functions; prevents and alleviates constipation (a natural laxative); the alkaline/acid balance, stimulates the appearance of new cells in the organism, as well as the metabolism of minerals and carbohydrates; induces rest, prevents deposits of calcium stones in the gallbladder and kidneys and helps the growth of bones.

**Problems caused by deficiency:** racked nerves, mental confusion, depression, irregular heartbeat, accelerated pulse, coagulation in the brain and heart, lack of appetite, diarrhea, nausea, improper nutrition and arteriosclerosis.

**Food that contains magnesium:** soy beans, legumes, bran, germinated wheat, whole wheat, wheat bran (raw), whole grain rice, whole barley, yellow corn, walnuts, almonds, all seeds, raw egg yolk, dairy products, Gruyere cheese, leaf vegetables, limes, grapefruit, oranges, apples, figs, peaches, mangoes, papaya, coconut, dry fruit and honey.

**Herbs that contain magnesium:** alfalfa, garlic, aloe, cayenne, dandelion, ginger, common comfrey, hops, great mullein, rosemary, valerian, chamomile, gotu-kola, parsley, peppermint, red clover, and seaweed (focus vesiculosus).

## Manganese

A trace mineral that is a component of enzymes involved in the synthesis of fats. Manganese is important for normal growth of bones. It is useful in forming thyroxine, for the metabolism of carbohydrates, and vitamins, particularly vitamin E, as well as supporting vitamin C and B without suffering any changes. It also assists in the manufacture of sexual hormones.

**Destroyed by:** too much milk, meat, calcium and phosphorous.

**Helps:** the central nervous system, to digest and to assimilated properly foods, recover energy, increase physical resistance, strengthen the muscles (and coordinate thinking with action), tissues and memory (improves the memory), as well as reproduction, breast feeding, diabetes and production of fatty acids.

**Problems caused by deficiency:** the development of bones and cartilage, as well as dizziness, poor memory, hearing (buzzing, noises) and lack of support to remove excess sugar from the blood flow.

**Foods that contain manganese:** legumes, green beans, whole cereals, corn, raw egg yolk, pecans, and green-leafed vegetables. Watercress, mint, parsley, celery, beetroot leaves, beet, sweet potatoes, bananas, bilberry, fresh fruit, dry fruit, and prunes.

**Herbs that contain manganese:** garlic, barberry, cascara sagrada, chickweed, horse tail, seaweed (focus vesiculosus), hops, yarrow, licorice, sarsaparilla, aloe, chamomile, black nut, and red clover.

## Molybdenum

A trace mineral that is a component of some enzymes. Molybdenum releases iron from the liver where it is stored, so that it may carry out its function of taking oxygen to the tissues and the cells. It collaborates with enzymes, helping them to eliminate toxic nitrogen waste and turn it into uric acid that it is then expelled from the organism as urea. Whole food contains sufficient molybdenum and the body does not need much. Excessive consumption may cause copper deficiency, afflictions of the bones, and gout.

**Foods that contain molybdenum:** legumes, beans, whole grain, and dark green-leafed vegetables.

## Potassium

Potassium and sodium work together to maintain the balance of several functions, such as that of the body's liquids and the conductivity of the nervous system. Potassium works within cell walls and mobilizes waste, nutrients, etc, through cell walls. Sodium plays its part outside cells. Potassium and sodium contain an electric charge expels waste form the cells and injects nutrients into them. Potassium, sodium and chloride maintain the balance of acid-alkaline fluids (organic), and the heartbeat.

Potassium is very alkaline and the organism eliminates excess through the kidneys and retains sodium. It favors digestion and the assimilation of food. Muscles and nerves contain a large quantity of potassium. Its influence may be seen in glandular functioning. Its daily intake should be between 3 to 4 grams in a normal diet. The body looses potassium when it subject to stress, either mental or physical, in cases of hypoglycemia, during long periods of fasting and because of diarrhea.

**Destroyed by:** processed food, and refined food such as flour and sugar, diuretics, coffee, and alcohol.

**Helps to:** transport oxygen to the brain, and nutritive substances to the cells; activate the liver, convert glucose into glycogen, remove waste, and helps the digestive system and secretion. It maintains the balance of sodium, in cases of tumefaction of the skin (edemas), maintains a good mood with grace and beauty, and keeps the muscles flexible and tissues elastic.

**Problems caused by deficiency:** hypertension, hypoglycemia, nervous system, insomnia, cardiac weakness, muscular and general weakness, edema, dry skin, thirst, constipation, gas, indigestion, buzzing in the ears, difficulty in breathing, and cramp.

**Foods that contain potassium:** molasses, unrefined brown sugar, red tomato juice, and red tomatoes, potatoes, green-leafed vegetables, pumpkin, carrots, watercress, celery, bananas, (all citric fruits), apples, cantaloupe, peaches, apricots, papaya, raspberries, sunflower seeds, oleaginous products, chestnuts, seaweed, milk, whole grain, beans, lentils, and raisins.

**Herbs that contain potassium:** alfalfa, garlic, chamomile leaves cayenne, aloe, dandelion, juniper berries, common comfrey, chamomile, cascara sagrada, echinacea, ginger, fennel, seaweed (focus vesiculosus), great mullein, parsley, mint, peppermint, valerian, yarrow, bitter *castella tortuosa*, golden rod, bearberry, and black nut.

## Selenium

Selenium is an antioxidant and works together with vitamin E without being transformed. There are small quantities in the organism, approximately half of which is found in the reproductive organs. Men need more selenium as it is lost in semen. Consumption of selenium through food is 0.3 mg (230 micrograms) a day.

- "The hypothesis that the AIDS virus slowly deprives the body of the selenium mineral.... supplements of the nutrient could combat this disease."*

**Destroyed by:** processed food, and food high in fat, as well as stress, hemorrhages, and old age.

**Helps to:** keep the tissues elastic, activate RNA and DNA, and the heart, keep the muscles strong, as well as metabolism (in several functions, such as the synthesis of proteins in the liver and red blood cells). Helps the function of the enzymes, stimulates the production of antibodies, connects oxygen to hydrogen and acts against lung cancer.

**Problems caused by deficiency:** loss of energy and vigor, weak and painful muscles with pain when walking, pain in the heart, brain hemorrhage, skin problems and premature aging.

**Food that contain selenium:** yeast, bran, wheat germ, eggs, milk, seaweed, red tomatoes, onions, broccoli, and Brazil nuts.

**Herbs that contain selenium:** garlic, leather weed, lobelia, and red clover.

*Chemical Medicine Magazine, A.P. Atlanta, Georgia, USA, August 19, 1994.

## Silica

Silica is a very important mineral for the organism's resistance to disease. It is the organism's surgeon.

**It helps:** to keep teeth strong, hair shiny, and nails healthy.

**Food that contain silica:** barley, oats, figs, strawberries, spinach, lettuce, asparagus, and red tomato.

## Sodium

Sodium is a mineral needed by the cells (see potassium). It is important for the acid-base balance and the functioning of the nervous system. It adjusts the heartbeat and regulates the content of liquids in tissues. It keeps minerals soluble in the blood, particularly calcium. It is the base mineral of the stomach and of the joints. It has a concentration of 0.9% in the blood. Daily intake through food should be 15 grams. It is found in all natural foods and to obtain it you do not need to add table salt (sodium chloride). Excess consumption is related to high blood pressure, loss of potassium, and edema. Fruits and vegetables are low in sodium. As a diuretic it is recommendable to consume herbs due to their high content of electrolytes. It is lost through sweating, vomiting or diarrhea.

**Helps to:** digestion and fermentation and counteracts acidosis, normal growth, the nervous system, active function of the muscles, purification of the blood, rebuilding glands, ligaments and blood.

**Problems caused by deficiency:** affects the nervous system, neuralgia, cramp, gas,

Indigestion, low sugar levels in the blood flow, loss of weight, affects the heart, arthritis,

drying of muscles, mental apathy and loss of appetite.

**Foods that contain sodium:** found in the majority of food except for fruit; celery, carrots, beetroots, asparagus, green beans, turnips, cucumber, strawberry, papaya, figs, coconuts, seaweed, Gruyere cheese, milk, raw egg yolk, barley cereals wheat and oleaginous products.

**Herbs that contain sodium:** alfalfa, dandelion, parsley, fennel, salvia, rosemary, thyme, chickweed, hawthorn, horse tail, aloe, marshmallow, sarsaparilla, *castela tortuosa*, seaweed (focus vesiculosus), and lobelia.

## Vanadium

Organic vanadium is a trace mineral. The small quantity found in the body is vital and lasts long. The liver stores a small part. Its function is to try to avoid the accumulation of fats in the arteries by reducing cholesterol and triglycerides.

**Helps to:** avoid heart attacks, metabolize iron, develop red blood cells, prevent tooth decay, and keep the teeth, bones and cartilage strong.

**Problems caused by deficiency:** low red blood cells, triglycerides, and cholesterol.

**Food that contain vanadium:** all whole grains and seaweed.

**Herbs that contain vanadium:** seaweed (focus vesiculosus).

# Iodine

A trace mineral or oligoelement and a component of thyroid hormones. It is transported to the thyroid gland where it produces the thyroxin hormone that affects and helps metabolism and growth. Iodine is important for the proper functioning of the thyroid gland. It is recommendable that pregnant and breast-feeding women take additional iodine as iodine deficiency may cause cretinism in babies (a type of retardation, see your doctor). It is suggested to consume natural iodine, as a high intake of medicinal iodine would have a contrary effect. Consume iodine gradually to avoid problems with the thyroid gland.

**Destroyed by:** processed food.

**Helps to:** the nervous system and the brain; burns excess fat, regulates organic metabolism, prevents goiter, helps healthy teeth, skin, nails and hair; regulates cellular and glandular activity and counteracts and expels poison.

**Problems caused by deficiency:** overweight, obesity, lack of energy, cold hands and feet, palpitations of the heart, slow mental activity, arteriosclerosis, nervous weakness, and may decrease the metabolic rate and cause goiter (hypothyroidism).

**Food that contain iodine:** garlic, onions, seaweed, kelp, vegetables grown in iodine-rich soil, sea salt, clay, mushrooms, carrots, tomatoes, potato peel, pineapple, pears, dairy products.

**Herbs that contain iodine:** seaweed (focus vesiculosus).

# Zinc

Zinc is essential for all the organism's processes. It plays an active part in the metabolism of enzymes and phosphorous. It is found in small quantities in the body, most of which is in the bones and muscles, and the remainder in the blood, liver, pancreas, kidneys, skin, retina and male sexual organs (prostate), insulin, and seminal fluid.

Zinc uses copper as a form of fusion. It is an important mineral for men and women. The daily recommendable intake is between 10 to 15 mg. It forms over 80 enzymes that are vital for synthesizing proteins and nucleic acids. Therefore zinc deficiency affects growth, the reproduction of cells, the libido, defenses against infections and the health of the skin.

**Destroyed by:** contraceptives, processed foods, alcohol, and old age.

**Helps to:** together with vitamin B-6, relieve strias, baldness and diabetes, improves digestion, prevents white spots on the nails and arthritis, keeps the gums healthy, gets rid of acne, and stimulate mental activity and the synthesis of protein and DNA. It also reduces levels of cholesterol, maintains the alkaline-acid balance and helps the prostate gland. It may be used to reduce sneezing and it may also reduce cold symptoms if taken as soon as they appear.

**Problems caused by deficiency**: arteriosclerosis, stria, lack of growth, scaly and rough skin, inflamed acne and assimilation of vitamin A. It affects night vision and causes lack of appetite (total or partial), problems in the liver and spleen, anemia and poor development of the sexual organs.

**Food that contain zinc**: yeast, soy beans, wheat germ, wheat bran, seaweed, eggs, sunflower seeds, mushrooms, green-leafed vegetables, such as spinach, and other vegetables.

**Herbs that contain zinc:** garlic, common comfrey, aloe, burdock, dandelion, chickweed, eyebright, hawthorn, seaweed (focus vesiculosus), licorice, hops, rosemary, marshmallow, golden rod, and sarsaparilla.

## Vitamins and minerals that organs need to function properly.

| | |
|---|---|
| Brain and nervous system | Phosphorous, magnesium, and B-1, A, and C vitamins |
| Pituitary gland | Bromide |
| Hair and nails | Silica and zinc |
| Bones | Calcium, phosphorous, and vitamin D-2 |
| Teeth | Zinc and phosphorous |
| Thyroid gland | Iodine and B complex |
| Heart | Potassium and vitamin B-6 |
| Stomach | Sodium |
| Intestines | Magnesium |
| Muscles | Magnesium |
| Liver | Sulfur, iron, and zinc |
| Spleen | Fluorine and copper |
| Kidneys | Zinc |
| Suprarenal glands | Tin |
| Skin and circulation | Sulfur and vitamins E, B3, and B12 |
| Migraine | Vitamin B-12 |
| Nervous system | Vitamins B1, A, and C |
| Night blindness | Vitamin A |
| Conjunctivitis | Vitamin B-2 |
| Colds | Vitamins A and C |
| Hemorrhages | Vitamin K |
| Dental cavities | Calcium, vitamins A, C, and D |
| Acne | Vitamins A and B6 |

| | |
|---|---|
| Asthma | Vitamin D |
| Cardiac insufficiency | Vitamin B-6 |
| Gallstones | Vitamin A |
| Colitis | Vitamins A and C |
| Rickets | Vitamin D |
| Varicose veins | Vitamins K, C, and P |
| Cells | Vitamin E |
| Fertility | Vitamin E |
| Scurvy | Vitamin C |
| Diabetes | Vitamin A |
| Strength of the blood | Vitamin B-1 |
| | |

Authors note: Before taking any vitamin, mineral or herbs suggested in all these sections of the book, talk to your doctor.

# A Glance At The Body's Systems

## THE DIGESTIVE-INTESTINAL SYSTEM

The human body's digestive system comprises the mouth, the pharynx, the stomach, the small and large intestines and associated glands, including the saliva glands, the liver, the gallbladder, the pancreas, the anus, and rectum.

The digestive system swallows transports, and absorbs food. These processes are carried out by hormones and enzymes being secreted from the pancreas, spleen, liver and gallbladder and food is converted so it may be digested.

The function of the digestive system is to process food to convert it into carbohydrates, minerals, proteins, fats and other usable substances, so that they may circulate in the blood flow and be used by the body.

A proper diet provides food for the body at maximum efficiency. You should eat well and keep your body clean and healthy so that you may be healthy and happy.

Digestion begins in the mouth where the teeth, tongue and saliva glands (that are not only moisten food, but also provide enzymes) grind down food into small particles that form the bolus. When swallowing the bolus, the peristaltic movement of the esophagus sends it to the stomach. The stomach segregates the gastric juice of hydrochloric acid in two ferments, these being pepsin and the coagulum. Pepsin and hydrochloric acid turns starch into an absorbable substance and the coagulum ferments milk.

In the stomach, starch continues the transformation that saliva started and that gastric juice will complete in the small intestine (duodenum, jejunum and ileum). Pancreatic enzymes and bile are discharged in the duodenum. The content of the stomach and the small intestine are called the chyme.

Chyme is transformed along the intestinal canal by the effect of the pancreatic enzyme (segregated by the pancreas) that contains salts and enzymes that are important for digesting fats, starch, and albumin; the gallbladder segregates the bile that acts on protein-based substances, and carries out an important emulsifying action on fats, lipids and lypo-soluble vitamins, and another anti-putrefaction action on nitrogenized substances, and also reinforces the digestive process of the intestine. There are also millions of intestinal glands that segregate the enteric juice (whose stimulus is the presence of the chyme in the intestine). It is made up of a number of enzymes including erepsin, lipase, sucrose, amylase, maltose, lactose, and nuclease, whose function is to terminate molecular degradation during the digestive process.

The intestinal canal absorbs water and nutrients contained in the chyme, so that they may enter the blood stream through the numerous vessels of the intestinal mucus. Once in the blood flow, they come into contact with various cells and take nutrients to the liver. The liver also receives blood from the spleen. This is the digestion and absorption process. Waste material passes to the colon which is made up of cecum, the ascending colon, the transverse colon, the descending colon and the rectum. It is in the large intestine where the body's health is determined.

A slow and inefficient large intestine affected by the accumulation of hardened toxic material that is encrusted in the intestinal wall, as little or none peristaltic movement, will allow toxins to be present longer than necessary. These toxins may be ingested or develop by fermentation or putrefaction of undigested waste or waste not eliminated properly. Therefore, they go to the blood stream so that the lungs, skin and kidneys eliminate them, affecting other parts of the body.

The cecum absorbs nearly all water and reduces the chyme to a soft mass called feces. The walls of the intestine segregate a mucus that is used to lubricate the fecal mass that then passes from the intestine to the rectum through peristaltic movements. The removal of ferments and putrefactions is a function of the intestinal bacterial flora. These friendly bacteria synthesize valuable nutrients when digesting the portions of fecal mass found there. There is little bacterial activity in the small intestine.

The most common problems are: indigestion, constipation, gastritis, duodenal or gastric ulcers, insufficient digestion of proteins, carbohydrates and fat.

## CONSTIPATION

Constipation is a serious threat for health and vitality and causes 99% of illnesses.

What is constipation? Constipation is a major accumulation of hardened fecal material in the intestine. The effort to excrete hard feces (evacuation) infrequently (every four days or more) results in various problems: the pressure on the intestinal walls is increased, causing the formation of bags called diverticulum, which fill with fecal material (or in the appendix) where bacteria find a suitable medium for multiplying themselves, thus causing infection (diverticulosis or appendicitis). It also prevents normal circulation of the blood in the lower part of the body and forms hemorrhoids (anus) or varicose veins in the legs. If the stomach is pushed upwards, a little above the diaphragm, this will cause a hiatus hernia. Fecal material decomposed in the intestine is a medium for the propagation of parasites and microbes in the organism.

**The primary causes are:** deficient nutrition, consumption of refined or processed food or food low in fiber, lack of water; ignoring the need to excrete contributes to self-poisoning, a sedentary way of life, mental and emotional tension, and poisonous substances such as alcohol, tobacco, coffee, chocolate, and sugar.

**Effects caused:**　hemorrhoids, insomnia, rheum, tonsillitis, amnesia, anxiety, headache, insufficient or too much appetite, grinding teeth, salivating at night on the pillow, itching in the anus, colitis and inflammation of the appendix.

**To aid the digestive system:** Drink two liters of water a day, drink two cups of hot water before breakfast, eat fiber, coconut, prunes, and boiled apple before going to sleep, and take two spoonfuls of olive oil or psyllium seeds in hot water before going to bed, or otherwise vegetable broth, fruit (grapes, mangoes, cantaloupe, papaya, etc), and vegetables. Fruit and vegetables are purifying sources of food. Exercise. Have a set time to eat. Clean the colon to keep healthy and ensure correct elimination and assimilation (garlic expels and neutralizes undesirable bacteria from the colon). Eat quality food that contains sodium, potassium and organic magnesium in order to maintain the colon's electrolytic level. Pectin absorbs gases and stimulates the intestines.

**Food that are difficult to digest:**　fats, fried food, sausages, franks, etc., bread, creams, and sweets.

**Food that is easy to digest:** fruit and raw vegetables, seeds and oleaginous products.

**The need for fiber:** Fiber is mainly found in nature.

Majority of fiber forms the volume of soft fecal material and is dragged by the mechanical action of peristaltic movement, this being highly beneficial, particularly for people with high levels of cholesterol and triglycerides. Some fibers, such as mucilage and gum, may absorb up to 40 times their weight in water, decrease the appetite and keep the digestive canal clean of putrid and toxic elements.

There are seven forms of natural fiber: pectin, bran, lignin, cellulose, hemi-cellulose, gums and mucilage, each of which has its own function, either mechanical or nutritional. They are divided into digestible and indigestible, and soluble (in water) and insoluble.

**Pectin:** ideal for diabetics thanks to its low absorption. It removes and eliminates toxins and metals, reduces the risk of heart disease, renal stones, and gallstones, and helps to remove cholesterol. It is of valuable use during radiation therapy. It is found in all citric fruits (in slices), bananas, apples, beetroot, green peas, etc.

**Bran:** has a high capacity to absorb water (mainly gums and mucilage). Its activity is reflected in producing an abundant soft fecal bolus in the intestinal transit full of fat.

**Lignin:** considered as the best way of reducing cholesterol. It prevents the formation of gallstones in combination with biliary acid. It is useful for treating cancer of the colon, arteriosclerosis and multiple sclerosis. It is contained in red tomatoes, potatoes, beans, carrots, apricots, strawberries, whole grain and Brazil nuts.

**Cellulose**: indigestible; found in the peel of fruits and vegetables. Helps treatment of colitis, constipation, varicose veins and hemorrhoids and helps remove carcinogen substances from the wall of the colon. It is contained in pears, apples, carrots, broccoli, beetroot, green peas, runner beans, Brazil nuts, etc.

**Hemi-cellulose**: indigestible. It is one of the complex carbohydrates that absorbs a large quantity of water. It is excellent for reducing weight and alleviating constipation and cancer of the colon. It is contained in pears, apples, bananas, beetroot, cabbage, green leaves, whole grain and beans.

**Gums and mucilage**: both are useful for reducing glucose in the blood, and cholesterol. They reduce appetite and remove toxins. They are contained in seaweed, oats, beans, and sesame seeds.

It is important to include fiber with your diet. The lack of ingestion of fiber results in problems in the gastro-intestinal tract, metabolism, glucose, and increases cholesterol.

**Soluble** fiber is contained in vegetables, seeds, beans and lentils and has the particularity of trapping fats and carbohydrates in the intestine, thus decreasing their absorption and reducing the risk of cardiac affections, by reducing levels of cholesterol. Psyllium contains soluble fiber and mucilaginous properties, in other words, the gum of the seed grows when coming into contact with water, producing a bolus and giving volume to the material that travels down the intestine, encouraging peristaltic movement. It should not be eaten in large quantities as it will have a contrary effect.

**Insoluble** fibers are found in cereals, bran, wheat, and whole meal cookies. They increase the fecal bolus and serve as a type of "broom", as they soften the feces, thus facilitating mechanical intestinal movement.

The quantity of fiber to be consumed depends on the size of your digestive system. It is advisable to consume between 20 and 40 grams of fiber a day and to take on sufficient water. Fiber detoxifies and thus prevents cancer of the stomach, the rectal colon and the pancreas, and breast cancer and prostate cancer. As fiber is low in fat, it prevents heart disorders, such as high blood pressure, cholesterol and triglycerides. Fiber invigorates the intestine and alleviates irritable and inflamed intestines, colitis, diverticulosis, appendicitis, and problems in the gallbladder, hemorrhoids, and varicose veins. Fiber is low in sugar so it controls diabetes by reducing and stabilizing sugar in the blood. You should include fiber in your diet. Insufficient consumption of fiber results in problems in the gastro-intestinal tract, with metabolism, glucose and also increases cholesterol.

Eating sufficient fiber in various forms, such as whole oats (ground) and beans (not soy beans), reduces cholesterol. Vegetables, such as carrots, cabbage, apples, green peas, etc., and wheat bran reduce polyps and improve regularity of excretion. Do not waste calories on food that does not contain fiber!

**Spastic colon:** (sporadic excretion, contracted and tense colon): eat carrots, beetroot and steamed whole grain rice, potatoes and pumpkins, sweet potatoes and bananas; chew and salivate well. Eat apricots and apples in syrup without the peel and the core. Drink vegetable juices, olive oil and eat yoghurt.

**Excretion:** place an object 15 cm high on the floor in front of the toilet in order to raise your legs. Raise your arms and turn your body. Massage your knees. If fecal material is thin, the colon is inflamed. If it is thick, there are too many proteins and fats and there is not enough fiber. Normal excretion must be abundant, compact, cylindrical, bronze, even and free of bad odor. Fecal material should come out all at once and float.

**Signs of dirty colon:** bad breath, body odor, and bad odor of excreted material.

**Causes problems with:** the prostate, the ovaries and/or womb, digestive system, liver, gallbladder, chronic disease, and acne.

**Flatulence and gases.** Cause by kidney infections, and excess mucus.

**Cleaning the intestine:** place one spoonful of flaxseed in a glass of water, leave to soak overnight, blend and drink before breakfast; or one glass of orange juice with three prunes (soaked) and two spoonfuls of sesame seeds, blend and drink before breakfast. Eat beet and beet leaves, cantaloupe, and steamed celery for 24 hours.

The intestine should be washed thoroughly using the colonics invented by Dr. Bernard Jensen. He says that colonic is vital as the intestine drastically spreads toxins throughout our entire organism.

What is a colonic? It is a gentle way of cleaning the colon by filling it with water at body temperature while lying down and relaxed, and then emptying it. It is not painful.

**Digestive problems caused by change in eating habits:** depurative crisis: the metabolism accelerates so you should take exercise, and brush your body.

**Excretion channels:** the colon, urinary tracts, skin (sweat), respiratory tracts (mucosa). The more congested the organ, the more it has to work.

**Detoxification:** gases and flatulence, headache, tiredness and anxiety, initial swelling of the system, semi-liquid or runny feces, may increase weight. In order to neutralize gases take a digestive or pancreatic tablets and to support the liver take beetroots and alfalfa tablets or cardamom tea. During a curative crisis, eat little or do not eat at all. Take on light liquids such as vegetable broth. If you have a fever, eat potato peel broth, and do not eat citric fruit. Drink sufficient water with chlorophyll or alfalfa tablets, and apply enemas. Look after all excretion channels.

**Intestinal hygiene:** Intestinal flora is made up of organisms that live in the intestine. This microscopic life includes a wide variety and it plays an important role in both health and sickness. Intestinal hygiene or cleanliness is not a simple task. It requires effort, work and will to adopt new methods, such as fasting, enemas, colonics, depurative diets and massage. For many years it is has been recommended to take liquid chlorophyll to recover intestinal flora that rebuilds, deodorizes and neutralizes, plus the wonderful beneficial bacteria called Lactobacillus Acidophilus (black tea, chocolate, coffee and white sugar destroys these bacteria).

The lactobacillus acidophilus turns sugars into lactic acid, creating an acid environment in which pathogen microorganisms cannot live. They synthesize enzymes that are essential for metabolism, speed up intestinal movement, prevent putrefying bacteria, remove bad breath, increase absorption of minerals, and reduce the risk of cancer in the colon.

**Help for digestion:** citric fruits stimulate the acids of the stomach and peristaltic movement of the intestine. It is recommendable to eat one hour before meals. Drinking enough water throughout the day, increases the level of hydrochloric acid. Chili also stimulates the increase of enzymes and of hydrochloric acid in the stomach, and increases the flow of gastric juices.

They also contain a compound called capsaicin, and the hotter the chili the more capsaicin it contains. They have remarkable anti-inflammatory, analgesic, anti-cancerigenic properties and are excellent for the heart. They contain vitamins A and C, beta carotenes and flavonoids. Digestion improves if you eat an apple at the end of the meal. Eat beetroot with its leaves or drink red tomato juice.

**Colitis:** eat raw onion with yoghurt.

**Irritated colon:** eat two bananas with cardamom seeds.

**Prolapsed colon:** take on calcium, yoghurt and acidophilus. Take two spoonfuls of sesame seed oil a day before breakfast or before going to bed. Drink coconut water.

**Colon with putrefied waste:** eat yoghurt.

**Diarrhea:** eat peeled and shredded apple for two days, break the diet with whole grain rice cooked with mungo beans and ghee (clarified butter); drink date milk or mint tea with onion juice every hour.

**Inflammation:** drink cucumber juice.

**Irritation:** eat apple boiled with cinnamon and a slice of lemon peel and honey.

**Ulcers:** drink celery juice with carrot. Eat red cabbage salad.

**Stomach:** eat raw fruit in the morning.

**Worms**:  drink papaya juice. Take one spoonful of fresh shredded coconut and one spoonful of castor oil two hours later.

**Parasites**:  papaya seeds remove all types of intestinal parasites. Take dry and crushed seeds taken with honey (20 grams for adults) and take castor oil two hours later.

**Indigestion**:  when you eat too much of something you feel that you have a ball in the stomach that sticks to it; this is improperly digested food. Small balls may also appear far from the abdomen in the ganglia, which should be massaged until they disappear. The symptoms are: not feeling well, not eating, and exhaustion. Drink hot mint or thyme tea or something frozen. Gently massage the ball with oil or herbs, pull the muscles of the spinal column and purge.

**To purge the liver:**  drink acidic juices: lime, sour orange, yellow orange, grapefruit, pineapple, cantaloupe, prickly pear, grapes, mango, capulines , artichoke, cayenne (piquín chili), olives, olive oil, carrot juice, celery, apples, lettuce and parsley. To detoxify the liver, apply enemas of coffee while fasting.

**Food that should be eaten raw:**  papaya, pineapple, cherries, peaches, prunes, shredded coconut, corn with starch, wheat germ, pumpkin, carrots, beetroots, cabbage, celery, beetroot, green-leafed vegetables, vegetable broth, lime juice, apple vinegar, bee's honey, olive oil, and yoghurt.

**Practical help for the digestive system**: do not drink liquids during meals (even less so with ice). Chew your food and eat slowly. Avoid fried food as much as possible. Try to fix a set time for eating. Eat in a pleasant environment and relax. Eat only what you need to satisfy your hunger.

**Practical support for the intestinal system:**  eat food with fiber. Exercise moderately every day. Go to the toilet when nature calls. Drink sufficient water or juice between meals. Avoid tension and dress comfortably with loose clothing.

## HERBS

**Carminative (gases):** sweet basil, cumin, fennel, chamomile, and cardamom.

**Anti-parasites:**  garlic, epazote, mugwort, chicory, male fern, *castella toruosa*, marjoram, black walnut peel, absinthe (in moderation), common clove. Tapeworm: pomegranate bark and root (purges in fasting). Worms: cinnamon and thyme taken together.

**Diarrhea:**  guava tree leaves.

**Constipation:**  fenugreek, ash tree, flaxseed

**Astringents:**  cranberry, plantain, marjoram and oregano.

**Infectious diarrhea:**  chamomile tea, geranium, and mint.

**Laxatives:** tamarind, chicory, fleawort, licorice, aloe and golden seal.

**Smoothing agents:** dandelion root, licorice roots, catnip, fennel, chamomile, great mullein, American elm, magnesium and calcium.

**Relaxing agents:** chamomile, mint, lobelia, and catnip. B complex vitamin and magnesium.

**Appetizers:** angelica, cumin. Appetizing and invigorating: rhubarb tea, aloe, and gentian._

**Stimulants:** ginger, piquín chili, cayenne pepper, beetroot, cinnamon, cloves, saffron, and mint oil.

**Peristaltic stimulants:** cascara sagrada, aloe vera (sabila), black walnut, alfalfa, barberry, red pepper, piquín chili, and oat bran.

**Spastic:** flaxseed, psyllium, marshmallow, great mullein, common comfrey, and licorice root.

**Depurative:** horse tail.

**Bad breath:** everlasting flower and/or chamomile with St. John's wort (homeopathic Hypericum) take before meals.

**Ulcers:** cuachalalate (*Juliana astringents*), balsam, celery, and golden seal.

**Digestive:** anis, honeysuckle, mint, rosemary, rhubarb root, aloe vera, chicory, verbena, boldo, cinnamon, *castela tortuosa*, quassia wood, dandelion, geranium, golden seal, marjoram, oregano, barberry, sunflower, cayenne, piquín chili, thyme (stimulates pancreatic enzymes), lemon balm, rosemary, chamomile (regulates stomach secretions), alfalfa, aloe vera, acanthus, fig, mugwort leaves, heliotrope, angel herb, white horehound, brickel bush, lime tea, English marigold, tlalchichinole, blackberry, muicle, mesquite, yellow elder, clover, golden seal, papaya, and ginger root contains the main active elements of ginseng.

Liver: the liver of people who are upset, anguished, or unsociable works deficiently. Drink sour orange, beetroot, dandelion root, beetroot, angelica root, horse tail, birch leaves, holy thistle, liverwort, parsley, barberry berries, burdock, Pau d' Arco, aloe vera, bearberry, golden seal, rhubarb, chamomile, absinthe (a little), oat bran, sodium (organic), and iron.

Milk thistle is used for treating gallstones, hepatitis, cirrhosis, psoriasis, fatigue, intoxication by medication, lupus, etc. seeds encourage the regeneration of the hepatic tissue.

**To reduce inflammation of the liver:** make a tea comprising: brickel bush 2%, boldo 4%, gram grass 10%, lime tree bark 3%, Castilleja 3%, scale fern 5%, artichoke 4%, quassia stem 4%, may be taken on their own or together.

**Spleen:** yellow orange (the same herbs as for the liver). Licorice root provides the spleen vitality.

# RESPIRATORY SYSTEM

The respiratory system comprises the nasal and frontal sinuses, the nasal passage, the pharynx, the larynx, the trachea, the bronchi, bronchiole, alveoli, and the lungs. All these tracts transport air to the lungs from where oxygen passes to the blood and carbon dioxide takes the reverse route.

Its function is to oxygenate, filter, moisten and heat the air that is breathed, and to keep the tracts free of foreign material. Lungs are covered by a membrane called the pleura that is lubricated by small quantity of liquid that allows the free movement of expelling and depressing, without causing pain during breathing. Lungs retain and concentrate energy. The main function of the internal organs is to produce energy and send it to the circulatory system.

The respiratory system is also a means of elimination through secretion. It has defensive mechanisms that comprise sneezing and coughing, which keep the tracts clear from foreign bodies. Oxygen is the base of life and protection of the system is very important. The lymphatic system is related to the circulatory and immunity systems. Nutrients and herbs that are used for the respiratory system are also used for the lymphatic system, as the mucosity produced by the lymphatic system covers the respiratory walls and sometimes causes congestion problems.

**Most common problems:** colds, flu, tonsillitis, influenza, coughing, bronchitis, asthma, mucosity retained in the body and inflammation of the cervical ganglia. Tobacco is involved in 90% of degenerative problems, chronic inflammation and deficiency in vitamins A, B, C, E, calcium, zinc, and magnesium.

**For colds:** boil the peel of one lemon, two cloves of garlic, brown sugar or honey in one liter of water for five minutes. Remove from the heat and add the juice of seven limes. Take 3-4 times a day. Watermelon juice cleans the liver and prevents further mucosity from forming. Apply a poultice of eucalyptus leave on the throat and chest. Drink pineapple juice, prickly pear fruit juice, berry juice, and oat bran broth.

**Fever:** take ginger tea with bee's honey and massage your feet with almond oil or castor oil.

**Recovery:** date milk.

**Hay fever:** eliminate dairy products. Place few drops of liquid chlorophyll on the nasal sinuses. Take a large dose of vitamins A, C, E, B5 and B complex. Minerals: calcium, magnesium, potassium, and manganese. Take a little Bee's pollen. Drink carrot juice, prickly pear juice, watermelon juice, and grape juice. Before breakfast drink Aztec tea and take one spoonful of wheat germ oil, one spoonful of lecithin with juice and seven alfalfa tablets. Apple vinegar.

**Throat:** scrape the tongue and take propolis. You should include lots of fruit and vegetables in your diet.

To help the respiratory system: take moderate exercise daily and abdominal breathing exercises. Try to be in places with clean air, do not smoke and avoid breathing cigarette smoke. Avoid or limit the consumption of dairy products. Brush your skin daily. Try to keep your digestive intestinal system in good condition.

**Breathing:** between 6 a.m. and midday, either seated or on foot, breathe deeply through the nasal sinuses expanding the lungs and stomach, count up to seven at the same time, contract the abdomen muscles upwards and downwards, hold the air in your lungs seven times and exhale gently seven times. Slowly relax the contractive muscles, continue with another series until you complete five minutes. Respiration must be slow and with a regular and continuous action at your own pace.

The skin is the second lung. It absorbs a quarter of the oxygen that we need. Dry-brush it to stimulate, clean and exercise it to keep the pores open. Brush from the feet to the neck. Walking, swimming, twisting and inflection help the lungs to breath more efficiently. Placing four fingers below the belly bottom supports the respiration as it is the balance zone between "the planet and the cosmos".

## HERBS

**Expectorants:** fenugreek (cleans and decongests), borage, licorice root, maiden hair fern and mallow.

**Asthma:** willow, elder and sundew (homeopathic).

**Hay fever:** alfalfa, red pepper, common comfrey, fenugreek, garlic, lobelia, great mullein, myrrh, chamomile, licorice, time, white willow, ginseng, ginger, and pau d' arco.

**Pectoral:** white nettle.

**Polyps:** bloodroot.

**Bronchial infections:** horehound.

**Smoking:** involved in 90% of all degenerative, inflammatory and chronic problems and deficiency in vitamins A, B, C and D and calcium, zinc and magnesium.

**Others:** alfalfa, aloe vera, mugwort, holy thistle, bougainvillea, great mullein, acacia, licorice, mesquite, sage, clover, arnica, horse tail, sundew, (psychic sector, when lungs host abnormalities), eucalyptus, maguey, sunflower, thyme, verbena, sage, hot radish, black walnut, pepper, echinacea.

Drink a tea made from borage, linden and eucalyptus. Eat capulin, watercress, celery, garlic, beetroot, and hawthorn.

The main function of the internal organs is to produce energy and send it to the circulatory system. The lungs retain and concentrate energy. All illnesses have an energetic origin.

## THE CIRCULATORY SYSTEM

The circulatory system is made up of the heart, arteries, capillary veins and blood, and includes:

The arterial system in which red blood circulates.

The venous system in which blue blood circulates.

And the lymphatic system in which lymph circulates.

The function of blood is to transport oxygen and nutrients to the cells of the body and to take metabolic waste and carbon dioxide to the elimination organs. Thanks to this process, all the body's systems may be kept healthy with the right proportion of oxygen and nutrients. The purpose of nearly all systems is to help maintain the blood's biochemical balance. The main function of the internal organs is to produce energy and to send it to the circulatory system body. The heart is the body's strongest muscle, about the size of a fist and weighing between 340 and 400 grams. It is situated behind the sternum and halfway up the chest. The function of the heart is to pump (it pumps from 4.5 to 5 liters a minute) blood through the arteries, veins and small vessels distributed throughout the body.

The heart conserves and concentrates energy. The balance is principally between the heart (fire-thought) and the kidneys (will or production and action).

The blood is nourished by the substances that circulate in the lymphatic system. Lymphocytes (red blood cells in their condition of birth) are also found in the lymphatic system and become part of the blood flow. All arteries have osseous protection. Ramifications branch out from the arteries to irrigate the vertebrae. The seven cervical vertebrae have an orifice that forms a canal which has an artery on each side (the vertebral artery) that go to the brain, together with the other two arteries. The Wilis polygon is at the base of the cerebral circulation. The origin of migraine is circulatory.

Tiredness and weakness are caused by the blood not having sufficient mineral salt nutrients. Problems regarding skin, nerves, ovaries are due to the lymphatic system being dirty. The liver belongs to the lymphatic system and the digestive system. The task of the liver is to remove toxins from the blood flow. If we help the liver, we can improve our destiny.

When we eat meat, the liver absorbs the vibrations animals suffer. Older people's blood tends to be thicker.

**Most common problems:** poor circulation causes cold hands and feet, high or low blood pressure, cardiac insufficiency, hemorrhoids, varicose veins, loss of hair and loss of memory.

**To help the system:** eat green-leafed vegetables, beet or beetroot, berries (strawberries, raspberries, etc), oat cereal, raw sauces, olive oil, and butter (in moderation).

**Anemia:** the capulin, peaches, apricots, and limes.

**An iodine-rich diet** helps to clean the lymphatic system. Radish is high in iodine.

**High cholesterol:** eat oat cereal, psyllium, activated carbon, vitamin E and omega 3.

**To purify the blood:** eat garlic, alfalfa (reinforces the blood) parsley, lime, oranges (limes and oranges remove mucosity and acids), grapes (transform the blood completely) onions (people with ulcers or high blood pressure should eat in moderation), tofu and sarsaparilla.

**Food that helps to decrease high blood pressure:** kelp (seaweed), garlic, cantaloupe, watercress, Saracen wheat, (piquín and habanero chilies eaten in small quantities) ginseng (helps the circulatory system and heart), lecithin, limejuice (thins the blood), vitamins C and B3; minerals: calcium, magnesium, selenium and co-enzyme Q-10.

**Practical help:** take gentle exercise everyday. Reduce your intake of fat (animal lard, and margarine), do not smoke and do not inhale cigarette smoke. Increase your intake of fiber with mucilage (vegetables, fruits) and complex carbohydrates.

**To help the liver:** do not eat heavy food, fats, fish, meat, eggs, fried food, chemical products and animal fats, alcohol and coffee. Do not eat between meals and dine heavy meals before going to bed.

**To clean the liver:** drink warm water before breakfast. Eat beetroot and its leaves, carrot and/or onion. Go on a mono-diet of watermelon juice or melon juice. Drink radish juice (daikon) diluted in carrots. Take exercise and sweat. If your urine is red, your liver is not working properly. Go on a gentle diet. Eat fresh steamed artichokes, mangoes and oranges. Eat steamed vegetables with yoghurt and cottage cheese for between one to four weeks.

**To clean the gallbladder:** eat hot radish. If you have gallstones, take the same amount of carrot juice, celery juice and cucumber juice.

Blood tonic: carrot juice, beetroot juice, parsley juice and spinach juice.

# HERBS

**Anemia**: walnut tree leaves, nut bark and husk, watermelon seeds, sunflower seeds and pumpkin seeds, mungo beans sprouts, almond milk, tofu (make a sandwich of tofu, bean sprouts, onion and red tomatoes to take on iron).

**Anti-hemorrhages**: yarrow, witch hazel, nettle, jacaranda flower, plantain, oak bark, chicken herb and geranium.

**Circulation**: alfalfa, aloe, cactus, watercress haw fruit, lemon balm, chicory, horse tail, Montezuma bald cypress, muicle, holy thistle, white hawthorn, mistletoe (has very strong astral forces), piquín chili and cayenne.

**Heart**: betel (also helps the memory, chewed prevents tooth decay and cures ulcers and cold sore). External use: pulmonary congestion.

**For the normal functioning of the heart**: white horehound and barberry.

**Reconstituting**: Siberian ginseng, sorrel, burdock, iron, dandelion (purifies), alfalfa, betel, apricot, blackberry, cranberry, red cabbage.

**Cholesterol**: fenugreek.

**Depurative**: dandelion, bloodroot, common comfrey, sarsaparilla, chicory, barberry, plantain, birch (advised for curing drainage), horsetail, burdock, golden rod, red clover, Turkish rhubarb root, burdock root (*arctium lappa*), American elm bark, wood soil (*rumex acetosella*) an old remedy for tumors, (use moderately).

**Nasal Hemorrhage**: passion flowers.

**Hemorrhoids**: great mullein, mallow; eat steamed beetroot leaves with lime juice. External use: eucalyptus oil.

**Menstruation**: chamomile, rosemary, horehound, marjoram, oregano, parsley, ruen (ruda), and cumin.

**Varicose veins**: Indian nuts with witch hazel.

**Liver**: Milk thistle (very important), angelica root, dandelion root, beetroot, horse tail, chamomile flowers, parsley, black cohosh root, hepatic, birchwood leaves.

**High blood pressure**: kelp, garlic, lecithin, ginseng, nutmeg (in small quantities)

# NERVOUS SYSTEM

The nervous system has the most important responsibility in the body. The nervous or peripheral system is made up of all the nerves that connect the cerebral trunk and the spinal medulla to the rest of the body.

Due to it its function it is divided into two parts:

**Central nervous system,** that is made up of the cerebrum, the cerebellum, the oblongata and the rachidian nerves, the spinal cord, meninges, and ventricular system.

**Autonomous nervous system,** that is not controlled by the will, such as the peristaltic movement of the intestine, stomach contractions, glandular activity and contraction of the cardiac muscle.

The autonomous or vegetative nervous system is divided into two parts:

| Sympathetic nervous system: stimulant. | Para-sympathetic nervous system: |
|---|---|
| Dilates the pupils | Inhibitor. |
| Dilates the bronchi | Contracts the pupil |
| Increases glandular secretion | Contracts the bronchi |
| Accelerates cardiac activity | Decreases glandular secretion |
| | Decreases cardiac activity. |

The main center of the sympathetic nervous system is called the solar plexus or the abdominal cerebrum, because here the functions of the digestive system and the internal secretion glands, which segregate hormones, converge. Alternative medicine stimulates functions of the solar plexus using friction and cold baths on the stomach.

The functions of the autonomous or vegetative system are nutritional and reproductive.

| Nutrition: | Reproduction: |
|---|---|
| Digestion ----- Assimilation | Secretion ---- Excretion |
| Breathing ---- Circulation | Dissimilation |

The brain transmits everything that surrounds us (sensitive function) and it sends information to the muscles (motor function) that react appropriately. The brain needs carbohydrates to function correctly. These are converted into glucose, the fuel or source of food for the brain.

**Most common problems**: nervousness, gastric problems or obesity of nervous origin, uncontrolled irritability, emotiveness, insomnia, headaches, lack of concentration and lack of muscular coordination.

**How to support the system**: do not eat quickly, do not go on diets high in protein, or consume refined sugar, coffee, tea, stimulants, alcohol, and dangerous drugs of any kind. Eat natural varied food (fresh fruit and vegetables, grain and seeds, wheat germ and flower pollen). Avoid tension, rest and relax, exercise every day (swim walk, etc). Take time for recreational activities, keep a positive mental attitude. Breathe deeply and meditate (the spiritual need is as important as the physical need).

**Food that helps the brain**: seeds, nuts, olives, onions, wheat, whole grain rice, corn, oranges, red tomatoes, lettuce, piquín chili, red peppers, wheat germ, and flower pollen. The gotu-kola herb is a great help for keeping the endocrine and sexual glands in good condition, and it provides energy for the cerebral and nervous functions. Consume ginseng and gotu-kola together, an excellent combination for combating mental and sexual fatigue. Eat peeled red tomatoes with mint and soy sauce three times a day for one week.

**Insomnia**: wheat, ginger, lecithin, olives, bananas, half a glass of celery or cucumber juice, wheat bran tea, and a capsule of calcium with a glass of hot milk with bee's honey. Massage your feet with almond oil, or castor oil with garlic juice.

**Depression**: B complex vitamin, calcium, sodium, and pineapple juice.

**Anxiety**: vitamin C, magnesium, and potassium.

# HERBS:

**Sedative**: mint, parsley, valerian roots and flowers, mallow, lemon balm, and satinwood (neurasthenia).

**Depression**: chamomile, valerian, and betony.

**Cerebral tonic**: ginger root, arnica (and the spinal column), gotu-kola, (source of vitamins B1, B2, B3, B5, B6, potassium, magnesium and zinc), hop flowers, and rosemary (stimulant).

**Others**: White willow bark, barberry, thyme, sunflower, marshmallow, passion flower, white horehound, aloe, toronjil balm, capulin leaves, and groundsel.

**Teas**: linden flower, orange flower, and leaves.

**Anxiety**: ginger, wild lettuce, gotu-kola, lobelia, white oak, red pepper, passion flower, mint, black cohosh root, and hop flowers.

# DRUGS:

**Alcoholism**: Drink large quantities of fresh and natural grape juice to speed up detoxification. Alternate every two or three hours ¾ parts of carrot juice to ¼ part of celery juice, and ¼ part of carrot juice with ¾ parts of celery juice. You may also eat beetroot with steamed leaves and eat yeast for three days, even if you do not have any appetite.

**Hangover**: one cup of yoghurt with the juice of two limes, and ice.

**Depression**: valerian, catnip, black cohosh, chamomile, lobelia, and betony.

**Smoking**: Eat ½ a cup of raisins everyday, take breathing exercises, and drink alfalfa water or liquid chlorophyll.

**Drugs**: Massage your feet in almond oil or castor oil with drops of garlic juice.

**Damage to the nervous system**: drink a glass of hot milk with two spoonfuls of almond oil (organic) or olive oil and 1/8 of a teaspoon of curcuma, and sweeten with honey to taste, drink every night for five weeks.

# URINARY SYSTEM

The urinary system is made up of the kidney, the urethras, the bladder and the urethra. The function of the kidneys is to filter blood, clean it of waste products and to maintain the balance of its water, salts and acids. All blood passes through the kidneys several times a day to be purified. Urine transports waste products from the kidneys, urethras, bladder and urethra to the exterior. The skin is known as the third kidney, as it releases poisonous substances from the organism through small sweat glands, thus detoxifying the internal organs.

When born, man brings with him a capital of energy that he uses throughout his life, this energy being stored in the kidneys. Sleeping well helps to conserve this energy. Suprarenal glands segregate part of the sexual hormones in men and women and help to adjust levels of energy.

**Most common problems**: pain in the kidneys, retention of liquids and infection of the bladder.

**How to support the system**: drink carrot juice with spinach juice in equal parts. Drink watermelon juice with seeds, cranberry, citric fruits, apples, green vegetables, lime, coconut water, beetroot with its leaves, watercress, whole grain rice with mungo beans, celery, garlic, artichokes, haw fruit, blackberry, radish, turnip, tamarind, and kelp seaweed. Diuretic food: melon, watermelon and its seeds, grape juice and pineapple juice. Include in your diet vitamin C, complex B, magnesium, potassium, large quantities of pure water or juices between meals. Eat a moderate amount of highly protein-based food. Urinate when your body tells you to.

Keep your sweat glands open. Take gentle exercise everyday.

# HERBS:

Dandelion, corn hairs, horse tail, bearberry, chamomile, parsley, juniper berries, Siberian ginseng, dong-quai, yellow elder root, sarsaparilla, acanthus, mallow, damiana, chicory, marshmallow, sweet basil, geranium, maguey, alfalfa, sage, aloe, verbena, yarrow, hydrangea, fig leaves, bark of the wild cherry and peach tree.

**Tea**: corn hairs, pinguica, borage and linden in equal portions, or bearberry or uva ursi, pinguica, and heather.

**Diuretic**: thyme, scale fern, queen of meadow, licorice root, borage, bearberry, great mullein, mistletoe, birch, barberry, corn hairs, uva ursi, fennel, common comfrey, tamarind, sanguinary, parsley, marjoram, oregano, horehound, honeysuckle, golden seal or golden rod.

**Kidney stones**: barberry.

**Infection in the bladder and urethra**: prickly pear (nopal).

# IMMUNE SYSTEM

The immune system is the organism working in harmony (it does not concentrate on a specific part or organ of the body). It recognizes foreign bodies (bacteria, virus, parasites, etc) and destroys or eliminates them. It also provides the body the ability to maintain its biochemical balance.

It may be said that the immunity system is made up of vessels, ducts, capillaries, glands and lymph. The tonsils are found in the lowest section of the oral cavity and behind the nasal cavities are the adenoid vegetations, formations that are an integral part of the immunity system. The lymphatic nodules function as filters of the system and are located in the neck, under the arms, in the groin, and around the lungs and intestines. The lymphatic nodes produce defense cells (lymphocytes and macrophages) against bacteria and other microbes. We need a large reserve of nutritive elements to resist the attack of lethal viruses and mutations on the cells that cause degenerative diseases.

The immunity system activates defense mechanisms to protect the organism from damaging toxins and harmful bacteria. The system's strength lies in the lymphatic system, considered as part of the circulatory system because lymph (always circulating towards the heart) mixes with blood by means of the large lymphatic vessels through the lymph nodes, finally entering via the blood stream through the veins in the neck region. The fluid of the lymphatic system only moves by muscular movement. The force of gravity tends to accumulate lymph in the lower part of the body.

**Its most important functions are**: transporting certain nutrients throughout the body, particularly fat and distributing white blood cells or leucocytes that combat all types of germs. The platelets are responsible for coagulation of the blood and collecting the large particles that may not be absorbed through the capillary membrane.

The spleen is also a lymphatic organ that contains plasmatic cells that produce many antibodies. The spleen is the center that absorbs vitality.

**How to support the system**: leading a healthy life reinforces the quantity and activity of immunity cells. Take light exercise everyday. Reduce contact with toxic elements because they saturate the system. Do not eat quickly, eat natural food, do not drink contaminated water and do not ingest conserving elements, chemical substances or antibiotics. Keep your body clean outside and inside by adopting a positive mental and affectionate attitude towards people, and meditate on the spiritual side of life.

Eating refined sugar reduces by half the capacity of white blood cells to destroy bacteria. Eat wheat, barley, and raw foods, such as cauliflower, broccoli, asparagus, cabbage, carrots and pumpkin (cooked) Chinese mushrooms, such as shitake, maitake, and reishi (with a immune-stimulating action), apricots, peaches, grapes, apples, berries, such as strawberries, blackberries and raspberries, lime juice, lime peel, green vegetables, vegetable soup, garlic, barley, wheat straw, molasses and bee's honey. Eat yoghurt, kefir, fermented cabbage and miso. Look after your intestinal flora. Keep your mouth healthy. Rest to recover, renovate and detoxify the body.

Take vitamins A, C, E, and zinc, manganese, chrome, selenium, and germanium.

## HERBS:

Siberian ginseng, pau d'arco, dandelion, golden seal, piquín chili, yarrow, thyme, *castela tortuosa* and burdock. Echinacea stimulates the activity of the Thymus gland, and actives the production lymphocytes.

**Depurative of the lymphatic system**:  fenugreek.

## GLANDULAR  SYSTEM

The glandular system is made up of the posterior, intermediate and anterior pituitary lobes, the thyroid glands, the parathyroid glands, the thymus, the pancreas, the suprarenal glands, the reproductive organs, the medulla and the cortex. It is said that the pineal gland, the thymus gland and the spleen have endocrine functions.

A gland is a soft organ that produces secretions (powerful biochemical substances) called hormones, whose objective is to maintain the chemical balance of the blood, this having a major large influence on all body functions. Its effects on the sense organs are related to metabolism.

**There are two types of glands**: **endocrine**, that lacking ducts release hormones directly into the circulation, and **exocrine** glands that release hormones through ducts known as sweat glands or saliva glands. The internal secretion glands are the most important and vital organs of our body and act closely with the nervous system. Hormones intervene in or control growth, development, reproduction, weight, emotional response, adaptation, maturity and many other functions.

**The hypothalamus** is not an endocrine gland, but it plays a very important part in the glandular system. It is located above the pituitary gland and below the thalamus. It regulates, controls and stimulates, directly or indirectly, each activity of the body and mind through the pituitary gland. If we learn to control the hypothalamus with the right amount of liquids and food, and control our will and mind, all glands will work together to bring peace and inner tranquility.

**The pineal gland** is located between the cerebral hemispheres in the internal posterior region of the brain, in front of the cerebellum. It plays an important role in the human superior  mind's mental activities. It is the master gland. It controls the skeleton and sexuality. When this gland "awakens", it makes the Superior Inner Self more sensitive and prepares it for higher states of conscience.

"The pineal gland produces the melatonin hormone and the enzymes responsible for its synthesis from serotonin through N-acetylation and 5-metoxilation identified in the pineal tissue of the mammals". Gnong, William, F., Medical Physiology Manual.

The pineal gland is a super gland. It segregates the melatonin hormone that reaches its highest levels during sleep, and is called the hormone of "eternal youth and peace". It is the key to our biological clock. It is responsible for the sleep-awake cycle, for adapting body temperature to the rhythm of yearly seasons; it corrects changes in times and depression. It regulates the glandular system and is involved in sexual desire and in the immunity system. According to studies, all these studies on melatonin were carried out by the Italian Walter Pierpaoli and William Regerson, professor of the University of Richmond, Virginia.  "We age because the pineal gland ages", says Pierpaoli.

**The food for this gland is**:   yeast, physiological phosphorous, wheat germ, celery, spinach, alfalfa, and bee's pollen.

**The pituitary gland** is situated in the "Turkish chair" of the brain, a privileged place. It is the third eye. These master gland secrets growth hormones. It is divided into two parts: the posterior part helps to maintain the balance of liquids in the body by stimulating the kidneys so that they reabsorb water and keep the involuntary muscles well invigorated. The anterior part stimulates secretion of hormones of the thyroid gland, and the growth of many parts of the body.

The pituitary gland controls the production of hormones in other glands. If the pituitary gland gives incorrect instructions or orders, the body looses its balance. This is related to the womb and the pineal gland which is awakened by the pituitary gland. Physiological food is the same as that of the pineal gland.

**To help the gland**: bee's pollen, and alfalfa.

**The thyroid gland** is situated in front and to both sides of the larynx and of the first rings of the trachea. The thyroid gland is full of vessels or ducts through which water, blood and lymph circulate every fifteen minutes. During this process, all impurities deposited in the thyroid gland produce an iodine deficiency that causes disturbances in its natural function.

The thyroid gland has a powerful influence on growth and development of the skeleton and on circulation of the blood. It also stimulates sexual functions, improves the texture of the skin, smoothness of hair, and has an effect on energy or lack of energy. The thyroid gland secretes hormones to regulate the metabolism of the entire body and it needs energy to function properly. It has an influence on the emotions and on intellectual and physical capabilities. The parathyroid gland controls the metabolism of calcium, magnesium and phosphorous in the body.

There is a simple examination discovered by Dr. Broda Barnes, author of the book "hypothyroidism", as follows: take the temperature in your armpit every ten minutes before getting up. If it is below 97.8, it shows that you have low thyroids.

**How to help the gland**: seaweed, black walnut egg yolk, molasses, parsley, apricots, dates, plums, kelp, garlic, onions, sea salt, watercress, mushrooms, carrots, green tomatoes, potato peels, pineapples, pears, dairy products, and safflower oil.

**Hyperthyroidism**: common comfrey and complex B

**Hypothyroidism**: herbal potassium, red seaweed (rich in iodine).

**Herb**: Seaweed (focus vesiculosis / encinilla de mar).

The thymus is situated in the upper part of the sternum and its external part is formed by lymphatic tissue. The internal part, or medullar, contains lymphocytes and inside a thick reticulum contains clusters of cells called Hassal corpuscles. The thymus is part of the immunity defense system of the organism. It controls responses to infected or malign cells; it plays a key role in producing the cells of the immunity system and it segregates the thymosin hormone.

Apparently, any abnormality of the thymus has something to do with auto-immunity illnesses and in the hyperplasia of the thymus, such as disseminated erythematose lupus, thyroiditis, hemolytic anemia, myasthenia gravis, and rheumatoid arthritis.

**The thymus is supported by**: Siberian Ginseng, Echinacea, lime peel, bran, thyme, *castila tortuosa*, pearl barley and carrots. Minerals: zinc, selenium and chrome. Vitamins: A, E, and C.

**The pancreas** is a very important gland in which water, blood and lymph play a very important part. The pancreas produces pancreatic juice. It has millions of dispersed cells called Langerhan barren isles, which constitute the endocrine portion of the pancreas. There are two types of cells: the most numerous segregate the insulin hormone, and others produce glucagons. Both are protein cells. Insulin is directly injected into the blood and serves to regulate the metabolism of carbohydrates and sugar levels in the blood (it also has digestive functions). Glucagons stimulate the liver's enzymatic system and determine the conversion of glycogen into glucose.

It is a regulatory and complex system that guarantees the right discharge of insulin in order to counteract the effects of glucagons and other glycemic hormones, so that glycemia is kept at normal levels.

Degeneration of the cells that segregate insulin causes the disease called diabetes mellitus, characterized by the presence of glucose in the urine and the large quantity of urine excreted.

The level of glycemia is increased by a reduction in the use of glucides, therefore the organism better consumes a quantity of fats and proteins, wearing tissues and causing acidosis. One of the factors of diabetes is the excessive consumption of flours, sugars and refined products. It is very important to drink vegetable juices and distilled or magnetic water, as they help the pancreas to function efficiently.

**To help the pancreas**: licorice root, lime peel, bearberry, golden seal and juniper berries.

**Diabetes**: drink cactus tea with seven ribs; boil water and place the cactus in it. Drink before breakfast and in the evening (a recipe of the Evangelist, Eugenio Ruiz Hernandez from Tlaxcala). Drink avocado seed tea, cut, sliced, and dried. Groundsel (Cacalia descomposita) root (decreases glucose, drink only for five days). Yellow elder, damiana, golden rod, common comfrey, croton (of hepatic origin), macho rosemary, thyme, cactus –nopal-(regulates the pancreas), celery, avocado, artichokes, amaranth, and apples.

**Tea**: yellow elder 10g, damiana 10g, eucalypts 10g, groundsel 10g, satinwood 20g. Boil in two liters of water, let stand for ½ hour, strain and drink three times a day.

**The suprarenal glands** secrete adrenalin to prepare the body for action in response to conditions of tension. They are found on each side of the spinal column, at the height of the first lumbar vertebrae and next to the upper pole of the kidney, where they take the form of a small triangle. They are formed by cortexes and medulla and they have a different origin and functions. The cortex derives from the mydodermic tissue and the medulla originates from the nervous ectoderm.

Hormones that secrete cells in the cortex help to control the metabolism of proteins, carbohydrates and fats, and to produce sexual hormones (in men and women). They also influence and regulate the concentration of sodium, potassium, and the liquids of the body. It also helps to adjust levels of energy to meet special demands.

The cells that make up the medulla affect the automatic responses of the organism. They affect various metabolic activities, such as those of glucides, increasing glycemia. They stimulate the heart (when the heart beats faster, the suprarenal glands are the cause). They relax the bronchial muscle and inhibit peristaltic movement of the intestine. The effects of the adrenal medulla are similar to those that produce the general stimulus of the sympathetic system.

<u>To help the glands</u>:  Siberian ginseng and licorice root.

**The spleen** is located behind and to the left of the stomach and is mainly made up of a tissue called splenic pulp. It is connected to the stomach and to the left kidney by ligaments. The spleen does not have an excretory tract so it may be considered as a true internal secretion gland. Its role is to vitalize and digest. Its movement is contraction-expansion and it swells while food is being digested.

Its function is to filter blood, and remove impurities in the blood and all bacteria from the circulatory system. The spleen produces antibiotics and it contains plasmatic cells that manufacture many antibodies. Thee spleen depresses during constipation, thus affecting digestion and creating a toxic environment that affects the entire system. The spleen produces lymphocytes.

<u>The most common causes of spleen problems are</u>: drinking alcohol, unhealthy water, very spicy food and not drinking water when you are thirsty.

<u>Suggestions for care of the spleen</u>: eat light food only, such as vegetable soup or steamed vegetables; drink lots of liquids, such as lime tea sweetened with honey, and fruit juice for one or two weeks at least twice a year. Avoid all types of fat. Drink raw vegetables juice once a day. Olives are good for the spleen. Licorice invigorates the spleen. Drink between meals, and do not prolong consumption. It is healthy. When needed, apply enemas.

Herbs: barberry, and elecampane.

# REPRODUCTIVE ORGANS

Female gonads.  The two ovaries produce the ovules that segregate estrogen and progesterone. Estrogens are responsible for the inherent characters of the feminine sex and of the reproductive process. They also stimulate development of secondary sexual organs, such as the uterus, vagina, fallopian tubes, vulva, breasts and nipples. Other effects of estrogens manifest themselves in the distribution of fat in the body to form the feminine curves, the growth of body hair under the arms and in the pubis, and the growth of bones.

When ovulation is completed, the follicle turns into endocrine tissue that segregates the progesterone hormone. Its objective is to prepare the uterus for implantation of the impregnated egg, support gestation and instigate changes in the structure of the mammary glands for breast feeding. Hormonal imbalance is caused by the incorrect ingestion of nutrients and constant tension.

<u>To help the female gonads</u>:  proper eating:  Vitamins C, B6, and Zinc.

To strengthen the reproductive organs and to rejuvenate the body: In a glass container soak a cup of whole wheat for three days. Leave it in a cool and dark place. Drink daily for seven weeks, and add clean water every day.

Eat plums, papaya, and apricots, peaches, citric fruits, watermelon, pears, bananas, grenadines, dates, figs, raisins, beetroot with leaves and green vegetables, all seeds and almonds, tofu, salad dressings, sweet potato, and potatoes.

**Menstrual colic**:   drink ginger tea with cardamom everyday (optional) during and after menstruation, and four days before take a spoonful of raw sesame seed or before breakfast.

**Irregular menstruation**:   before eat eggplant, and during eat mango, and maintain a fruit, and vegetables diet.

**Abundant menstruation**:   lecithin and vitamin E.

**Menopause**: vitamin E, chlorophyll and crude oils (sesame, peanut, olive, coconut, almond). Wheat cleans and nourishes the intestinal tract, makes the skin attractive, strengthens the skin and gums, and prevents pain in the lower part of the back. Eat curcuma twice a day to increase sexual energy, clean the reproductive system and keep all mucus membranes in optimum condition.

Herbs: dong quai, red pepper, piquín chili, ginger, golden seal, queen of the meadow, holy thistle, black cohosh, red raspberries, damiana, and baneberry.

**Aphrodisiacs**:   sweet basil, and damiana.

**Irregular menstruation and excessive bleeding**:   golden seal.

**Vaginal washing**:   gold seal.

**Male gonads**. The male testicles produce and store spermatozoids, and produce the testosterone hormone that distinguishes the male sex: tone of voice, external conformation, hair on the face, etc. It also develops the secondary sexual organs: the urethra, prostate glands, scrotum, testicles, deferent ducts and the seminal vesicles in the penis. It also influences metabolism.

The most frequent problems of the male reproductive organs are those associated with the prostate gland. The most common disorder is inflammation (prostatitis). The causes are: infections caused by toxic processes and malnutrition, indigestion, constipation, long periods between urinating, consumption of alcohol, tobacco, and a sedentary way of life, and possibly due to excess or lack of sexual activity or masturbation. Its symptoms include pain, burning sensation or frequent desire to urinate in small quantities and a sensation of not having urinated completely.

**To help the male gonads**: zinc (a mineral associated with the functions of the reproductive system), nickel and copper. Herbal nutrients that clean, reduce inflammation, mineralize and regenerate the prostatic cell:  horse tail, Indian nuts, cypress, shad, and shepherd's purse.

One of the main causes of sexual dysfunction in men is caused by the stomach being full at meal times. A simple remedy is to go on a liquid diet for several weeks comprising juices and soups, followed by a normal diet with nutritional food, eating in moderation.

In order to strengthen the nervous system after having sexual relations and without resting drink sesame seed milk and ginger or warm milk with sesame seed oil.

Men should eat two cloves of garlic a day, as this stimulates the production of semen and strengthens sexual energy. Clarified butter and nutmegs (decrease blood pressure) are excellent for problems of premature ejaculation. Take one teaspoon of shredded nutmeg with yoghurt before having sexual relations; with banana it as excellent invigorating properties. Onions and saffron generate sexual energy, and increase the production of semen. Eat raw pistachio nuts without the husk and salt. Fruits: bananas, pineapple, pears, papaya, prunes, and peaches are all delicious when blended with yoghurt.

## HERBS:

Gotu-kola, Siberian ginseng, sarsaparilla, echinacea, saw palmetto, damiana, garlic, piquín chile, red pepper, and licorice root.

**Prostate gland and kidneys**: ginseng, yarrow leaves, woodruff, juniper berries, golden seal root, marshmallow root, red pepper, piquín chile, parsley, horse tail, cypress, Indian nuts, shad, and shepherd's purse.

**Aphrodisiacs**: sweet basil, and damiana.

**Common problems of the glandular system**: sterility, exhaustion or insufficient vital energy, lack of growth in children, metabolic problems and imbalance of hormones, caused by the lowering of defenses. Avoid tension, polluted environments, refined foods, drugs (cause drowsiness), alcohol, black tea and coffee. Do not overdo X-rays particularly in the pituitary gland area.

The main function of the internal organs consists of producing energy and sending it to the circulatory system.

**To help the system**: eat lecithin, asparagus, sesame seeds, sunflower seeds, pumpkin seeds, all types of oleaginous products, berries: strawberry, raspberry, etc, bean sprouts, alfalfa, carrots, turnips, beetroot, seaweed, seeds, and vegetable roots. Vitamins: A, E, C, B5.

**Minerals**: potassium, zinc, and manganese.

## HERBS:

Parsley, alfalfa, and thyme.

__Tonic__ herbs: fennel, damiana, dong-quai, and flower pollen.

__Hormonal__: common comfrey, dong-quai, holy thistle, epazote, damiana, oregano, sweet basil, alfalfa, aloe vera, chamomile, radish, and muicle.

__Roots__: dandelion, echinacea, ginseng, dong quai, and marshmallow.

# STRUCTURAL SYSTEM

The structural system is made up of bones, connecting tissues, muscles, membranes and skin, all of which constitute the form, structure and mobility of the body.

The osseous system is that which supports the weight of the body and acts as a handle that allows the body to move. It protects vital organs, it is a store of calcium and phosphorous and it forms blood cells. Muscles provide us the ability to move and they represent over 70% of our bodily weight. In order to keep muscles healthy you must keep a good diet and take frequent exercise, which also stimulates the nerves and blood and lymphatic irrigation. All the body's muscles are connected to the bones by connective tissue and keep the bones joined. Membranes (internal tissues) are those that protect the walls of the respiratory and digestive tracts. The skin, the third kidney, is very important; as it is an assimilation and elimination organ (it filters waste from the blood through the sweat glands). Skin problems may be caused by accumulated toxins, a result of the other elimination organs not doing their job properly; if other systems carry out their functions properly, the structural system will remain healthy.

__Common problems in the bones__: osteoporosis (demineralization), loss of elasticity of ligaments, lumbago and calcium deposits in the joints.

__Common problems in the muscles__: deposits of acid that when healing form gellos; tension, high and constant contraction, and insufficient strength.

__Common problems of the skin__: loss of hair, acne, eczema, cracked nails, and dries skin.

__How to support the system:__ Keep your digestive system in optimum condition, particularly as far as levels of hydrochloric acid in the stomach are concerned. Drink sufficient water between meals. Avoid refined foods, preservatives, and sodas. Do not eat meat, particularly if you are old. Exercise. Maintain a correct posture. Use neutral or balanced pH soap. Brush your skin.

Massaging prevents muscular tension, strengthens the structural system, allows the blood and lymph to flow properly and provokes a healthy response of the nervous system.

Drink carrot juice with raw potato, potato peel broth, coconut, ginger (relieves back pain); eat curry, whole grain rice with mixed vegetables: ginger, onion, ghee, curcuma, cloves, cardamom, black pepper, and cinnamon. Raw fruits in abundance: papaya, grapes, etc.; green-leafed vegetables; dairy products: butter (in moderation), yoghurt, cottage cheese and light cheese; nuts and seeds, whole and raw, millet seeds, whole grain rice, barley and oat bran. To **lubricate the joints**: blend one cup of hot milk, add a pinch of curcuma, two spoonfuls of almond oil, and honey.

**For the skin**: chamomile tea, lecithin, papaya, and grapes.

**Mono-diet**: boiled grains of wheat or green vegetables, and zucchini.

**Dry and scaly skin** (on the ears too) this may be due to a deficiency of phosphorous or other nutrients in the nervous system: banana, olives, coconut, and wheat germ.

**Nettle rash and mosquito bites**: calendula.

**Slight burns**: apply raw sliced potato. To get rid of eczema and warts, drink milky papaya juice, and apply. Apply vinegar.

**Minerals for the bones**: zinc, calcium, magnesium, copper, phosphorous, manganese, boride, all trace minerals, hydrochloric acid for unfolding and absorbing minerals, and proteins.

**Muscles, connective tissues and joints**: Vitamin C with bioflavonoid. **Skin**: zinc, silica, vitamin C with bioflavonoid, and essential fatty oils.

# HERBS

**Bones**: alfalfa, common comfrey, borage, and marsh mallow.

**Muscles**: alfalfa, chicory, sorrel, white willow bark, devil's claw, American elm, yucca, and great mullein.

**Skin**: for external use for washing: chamomile, calendula and willow flowers. Internal use: burdock. Skin and its problems are also related to the thyroid gland (5th generator): sage, black walnut, dwarf oak, sarsaparilla, curcuma, and barberry.

**Joints**: alfalfa, red pepper, piquín chili, valerian, sarsaparilla, white willow oak, lettuce, black walnut, yucca, black cohosh root, *castela tortuosa*, yarrow, hydrangea root, centaury, catnip, bromelin, American elm, and skullcap.

226

**Rheum**: sunflower.

**Hair**: rosemary, horse tail, seaweed, and horehound.

**Sweat glands**: borage with sarsaparilla, cinnamon with lemon, juniper, geranium, honeysuckle, eucalyptus, marshmallow, burdock, lemon balm, sage, elder, thyme, cilantro, and hazel.

**General weakness**: cinnamon, damiana, gotu-kola, parsley, mint, rosemary, thyme, arnica, oregano, white hawthorn (for the heart) Pau d' Arco (Taheebo), and raspberries.

**Author's note**: Before taking any vitamin, mineral or herbs suggested in this section of the book, talk to your doctor.

# The Advantages Of Some Herbs Mentioned In This Book:

**Wild chicory**: the leaves are invigorating, purifying and diuretic. Slightly bitter but pleasant with salads.

**Barberry**: helps for pulmonary infections and reduces fever; relieves problems of the circulatory system and removes obstructions of the liver, and gallbladder.

**Liverwort (agrymony)**: considered by Egyptians as a panacea. Rich in enzymes that help to clean the liver, and the circulatory system. Relieves problems of the kidneys and is diuretic. May also be used for afflictions in the mouth, and throat. External use: gargling.

Iodine seaweeds: these sea plants help to purify the blood, improve energy capacity, and rejuvenate the body.

**Absinthe**: very bitter. Take with precaution only for a couple of weeks. Reduces fever, is appetizing, digestive, and hepatic, facilitates menstruation, and removes intestinal worms.

**Angelica**: acts as a stimulant in the respiratory tracts, removes colic, and helps irritated stomach.

**Mugwort**: excellent for cleaning the liver, the gallbladder and kidneys, and may also be used to cure scratches and wounds. Cleans toxic waste from the mucus membranes in the bronchi, and helps digestive problems.

**Burdock**: helps to detoxify the organism, clean the blood flow, increase perspiration, reduce accumulation of water and tissues and cells, it is said that it cures tertiary syphilis. External use: apply a poultice of the fresh root on warts.

**Boldo**: grows in Chile, it is bitter and has a strong antiseptic power. Excellent for the liver, and the genital-urinary system.

**Borage**: its name in Arabic means "father of sweat". It is used as a medicinal plant and as a vegetable. Helps relieve inflammation of the respiratory tracts.

**Calendula**: or "marvelous" that helps remove obstructions of the liver, and menstrual problems.

**Cascara Sagrada**: a natural laxative.

**Indian nuts:** help to strengthen resistance of the blood vessels, and to heal hemorrhoids.

**Horse tail:** a great source of storage of silica; therefore it is a great re-mineralize. Helps to combat rackets, and helps to join fractured bones, may also be used against urinary incontinence. and urine with blood in it.

**Common comfrey:** a plant that is capable of joining bones. Acts as an emollient and expectorant in cases of bronchial problems. Helps regeneration of gastric mucus (ulcer). External use as a compress: for healing burns and small wounds.

**Dandelion:** its enzymes help to detoxify the liver.

**Juniper:** helps to stimulate slow processes, and is useful as a natural diuretic.

**Hawthorn:** the infusion of dry fruit acts as a diuretic and to relieve diarrhea. The branches' bark helps to reduce fever. The flower stabilizes and combats tachycardia. Acts as a stimulant of the heart, and eases problems of blood pressure. Helps clean accumulated incrustations.

**Eucalyptus:** helps reduce fever, relieves influenza and bronchitis, calms asthma and destroys bacteria.

**Fenugreek:** contains mucilaginous enzymes that help inflamed digestive organs. As a poultice it may be used for wounds, and inflammation.

**Gentian:** helps against dyspepsia and digestive problems.

**Geranium:** (or the San Roberto herb): decoction efficiently relieves gastric ulcers, internal hemorrhages, gastroenteritis, and diabetes. External use: make a poultice of crushed leaves to remove obstructions from the breasts of breast-feeding mothers.

**Ginseng:** this root is very appreciated by the Orientals due to its high content of enzymes; it is used for healing everything. It is a powerful restorer that supposedly prolongs life and acts as a natural aphrodisiac.

**Great mullein:** the flowers and leaves relieve colds with a calming action. It is said that it attacks harmful bacteria that cause infection. In Ireland it is taken boiled with milk to cure tuberculosis. External use: as a poultice to cure abscesses and warts; the juice may be drunk to provide an efficient purifying action.

**Peppermint:** its enzyme helps to remove gas and intestinal spasms, according to herb experts; it helps to cure the gallbladder, and kidneys with its diuretic action.

**Catnip:** relaxes the digestive system, and reanimates the circulatory system, creating a sensation of well being.

**Fennel**: helps to relax nervous stomach disorders.

**Ginger** (wild): strong roots that act on the kidneys to help wash viscous accumulations and to improve hormonal function. Provides resistance against respiratory diseases.

**Lavender**: it has always being used as a powerful antiseptic. Taken as a tea three times a day it removes migraine, helps difficult digestion, and cures flu, asthma, and bronchitis.

**Flaxseed**: the gummy seeds should be soaked before eating. It may be used against afflictions of the intestine, and to remove toxic accumulations. This is useful for the bronchi, kidneys, and the circulatory system. External use: apply a hot flour poultice in cases of bronchitis, and muscular pain. Prepare when needed because if not properly preserved it produces hydrocyanic acid, causing skin rashes.

**Lobelia**: useful for curing respiratory problems such as asthma, and bronchitis. External use: use as a poultice on twists, inflammation, cuts, and wounds.

**Mallow** (great and small): cures bronchitis and calms inflammation of the urinary tracts. External use: gargling.

**Marshmallow**: cures abscesses, warts, irritation of the skin, and mucus. External use: gargling.

**Chamomile**: a panacea. It removes colic and gas in the intestine, facilitates digestion, attenuates gastric spasms, returns the appetite and helps in the assimilation of food. It may be used against general fatigue. It facilitates menstruation. External use: skin ulcers, twists, inflammation of the eyelids, etc.

**Mint**: the leaves and flowers help to weaken mucosity in the bronchi. It is a digestive and calming tonic, and removes gases.

**Mistletoe**: grows on poplars and apple trees. It is considered as a panacea. Excellent against arteriosclerosis, and hypertension. Rudolf Steiner uses it as a therapy against cancer.

**American elm**: when you chew the inner bark a bland mucilaginous enzyme is released that acts as an emollient, removing coughing spasms. External use: this bark of young branches may be cooked, and applied as a compress on eczema of the skin and herpes.

**Passion tree**: of special use for the nervous system, insomnia, and anxiety.

**Parsley**: the entire plant is a source of curative enzymes. Alleviates inflammation of the internal organs, and reduces intestinal gas. Help the bladder.

**Licorice**: its roots are sweet, moist, and mucilaginous. Helps against problems of excessive acidity and acts as a sedative of the irritated mucus membranes of the bronchi. Improve the blood flow.

**Rosemary**: a natural tonic against headache that also helps the hair grows, and acts as a stimulant of the circulation. Its magical power is protective.

**Rhubarb**: (do not use the leaves as they are toxic). Drink tea made from its veins in small quantities as an energy-giving drink. If the dose is increased it becomes purgative. Drink prudently.

**Elder**: all of its parts are used, the fruit as a laxative, the leaves are diuretic and purifying, the flowers are used against influenza and children's illnesses, and the bark helps against hydropsy.

**Linden**: calms the nervous system and may be used to alleviate insomnia, headache, palpitations, and anguish.

**Red clover**: the flowers are of a red-pink color and their enzymes help to purify the blood flow and improve the production of red, and white blood cells.

Laboratory analyses and tests show very important concentrations of substances called isoflavones that are similar (but not identical) to estrogen, although the effect of these phytoestrogens is very gentle. Clover's isoflavones include soy, genista, daitzein and cysteine that are relevant in hormonal problems of women, and of men to a lesser extent. It seems to regulate cycles, anguish, and depression, removes redness of the skin, is effective against cancer and leukemia, and is a general detoxifier.

It is well known in Europe for treating radiated patient or those subject to chemotherapy.

Doctors, naturists, and herb experts use clover efficiently for pre- and post-menopausal problems, as it purifies the blood, and against tumors, etc.

It contains vitamins A, C and complex B, proteins, minerals, iron, molybdenum (a trace element that is very important for removing nitrogenous waste; it also acts as an accelerator, together with iron, in the production of antibodies).

**Thyme**: its enzymes help to clean the bronchi, calm spasmodic and irritating coughing and eliminate intestinal gas. Thyme used to be burnt and inhaled as a means of self-cleansing.

**Valerian**: a powerful tranquilizer of the nervous system in cases of epilepsy, depression, hysteria, migraine, convulsions, and cramp.

**Verbena**: the druids considered it having magical properties. Taken as a tea it helps pregnant women to invigorate the uterus and breast-feeding mothers to increase milk. External use: apply as a poultice for sciatica, and lumbago.

**Fleawort**: decreases inflammation and helps to remove accumulations in the bronchi-stomach-intestinal systems. Its seeds often form the basis of laxatives.

**Blackberries**: the whole plant may be eaten. It is an important source of enzymes that boost the action of citric and malic acids that help to clean tartaric deposits in the mouth and teeth, and in some organs of the body.

**Sarsaparilla**: originated in Mexico. It is diuretic and purifying and helps to clean the circulatory system of toxic waste. External use: apply as a poultice to reduce inflammations on the body.

# A Glance At Ecology

Nutrition and ecology are closely linked; they are life itself. Many people are very concerned about the precarious situation of the environment, brought about by a reduction of the earth's resources and overpopulation, and they provide solutions. The answer could be simply to reduce the amount of meat we eat. There would be sufficient food for every man, woman and child in the world and is probably the simplest, most significant and most powerful thing that we can do, to avoid the destruction of our environment and conserve our precious resources. It is a simple matter of economizing.

Millions of acres around the world have been deforested for pasture and for breeding animals (basically livestock) and half farming land is used for feeding animals. Therefore, an enormous number of plants, needed to feed the human race, are used for feeding livestock at a high cost of transforming forage into meat.

To produce one kilogram of meat, a cow needs to eat 16 kg. of cereal, soy, and forage; drink 9,500 liters of water and use energy equivalent to four liters of gasoline. To produce one kilogram of meat, a chicken needs to eat 3 kg. of food and drink 1,578 liters of water.

Frances Moore Lappe, a French nutritional doctor, has given us a very significant example. When one eats a 225 g. steak, 45 or 50 people could eat a cupful of cooked cereal and soy. Ninety percent of this protein is wasted by "recycling" the grain through livestock. If consumption of meat was reduced by 10%, the extra grain would feed many people and hunger would no longer be a problem. "Malnutrition is the disease of injustice".

Grain and soybeans are excellent sources of protein and their nutritive value is used much more efficiently when consumed by man. Let's take interest, let's provide support, and let's provide the place that the farmers of the modern day deserve; so that they continue loving nature, instead of seeing it in terms of profits. What nostalgia for nature and day-to-day happiness!

## THE GREENHOUSE EFFECT

Cows contribute greatly to the greenhouse effect. "The millions of cows around the world produce millions of tons of methane a year, a powerful greenhouse gas that molecule by molecule traps 25 times more solar heat than $CO_2$". Animal excrement amounts to millions of tons a year (equivalent to the waste of half the world's population), therefore, excess manure and fertilizer ends up in the drains.

Georges Borgstrom, a specialist in the geography of food, believes that livestock contributes ten times more to the pollution of water than the human race does, and three times more than industry. Excrement in the soil is converted to nitrates, nitrogen, and ammonia, which filter through to underground water and surface water.

**The greenhouse effect.** The earth's atmosphere traps the heat of the sun as does a glass or plastic roof like those of a greenhouse. Sunlight heats the earth, but heat that is generated, spread in the form of infrared radiation, does not easily escape from the atmosphere. Greenhouse gases block radiation and return part of it to the earth, thus contributing to global warming.

## THE OTHER LUNGS OF THE PLANET

A number of photographs taken from the NASA Nimbus-7 satellite shows parts of the earth that produce oxygen and remove carbon dioxide, due to phytoplankton.

Phytoplankton contains chlorophyll, (that makes photosynthesis possible, comprising the formation of organic molecules from inorganic molecules). It absorbs sunlight and allows these minuscule plants to remove carbon dioxide from the atmosphere that it enters and is dissolved in water, to fix it in the form of carbohydrates to its biological structures.

Phytoplankton are green-blue algae that contain other photosynthesizing pigments (autotrophic bacteria), different from the chlorophyll that fix carbon and expel oxygen. It is found more in coastal areas than in the depths of the ocean. When plants die, they take carbon to the ocean bed. Phytoplankton renews itself more quickly than animals in the ocean that eat it. It is a basic source of food on which everything depends, directly or indirectly. It is subject to changes of season, and depends on light and nutrients, such as seas threatened by pollution that reduces population.

## STATISTICS ON HUNGER.

1.  Around 24,000 people die every day from hunger or causes related to hunger. This represents a decrease from 35,000 people a day ten years ago and 41,000 people twenty years ago. Seventy-five percent of people who die from hunger are children under the age of five*

2.  Nowadays, 10% of children in developing countries die before the age of five, a reduction of 28% when compared with 50 years ago*

3.  Hunger and wars caused just 10% of death by hunger (sic), even when these causes tend to be heard more frequently. Most deaths caused by hunger are due to chronic malnutrition. Families do simply not get enough food, due to extreme poverty.

4.  It is estimated that more than 852 million people in the world are affected by hunger and malnutrition, around ten times more than the number of people who die of hunger every year.

5.  Chronic malnutrition not only causes death, but also visual problems, lack of appetite, deficient growth and much greater susceptibility to suffering illness. People suffering from malnutrition are incapable of functioning even at a basic level.

6.  Many experts in hunger believe that at the end of the day, education is the best way of reducing hunger. People who have access to education have the best possible means to get out the vicious circle of poverty that leads to hunger.*

7.  Very often, only a few and simple resources are needed for poor people to be able to grow the food they need to become self-sufficient. These resources include quality seeds and the right sources of water. Farming and food storage techniques should also be improved.

* Sources: (by paragraph)

1) The Hunger Project, United Nations

2) CARE

3) The Institute for Food and Development Policy.

4) Organization of the United Nations for Agriculture and Food (FAO).

5) The United Nations World Food Program (PMA).

6) United Nations Children's Fund (UNICEF).

7) Oxfam

# DO WE KNOW WHAT TO DO WITH KITCHEN WASTE?  NO?

Then, let's talk about garbage.

We know that…

- It is difficult to accept that garbage is waste that we produce, in nature it does not exist as such.

- We live with garbage in our homes, streets, garbage deposits, etc.

- Everybody loses control of their own waste.

- We produce garbage by throwing away everything mixed up, thus attracting flies, rodents, cockroaches, etc.

All this contributes to pollution of the soil, waterbeds, jungles, seas, lagoons and the air (due to burning and bad odor).

We realize that

- We produce millions of tons of garbage every day (one kilogram per person per day) 60% being organic.

- Recycling excessive packaging will help to decrease the amount of garbage. This comes from the garbage store.

- Now is the time to make the change.

What we can do

- Reduce garbage by buying responsibly, preventing unnecessary consumption and accepting only returnable packages.

- Reuse (several times) plastic, glass, Styrofoam containers, etc.

Separating garbage into two types:

1. **Inorganic** garbage: industrial waste, including metal, glass, plastic, rubber (tires), various, etc. Washing and crushing all containers reduces their volume five times.

2. **Organic garbage:** originates from live organisms: fruits, leaves, grass, branches, bones, wood, paper, etc. This waste may be used to make compost.

# COMPOST

Compost is any type of vegetable that falls to the soil and uses oxygen as part of its natural putrefaction process.

There are several ways of making compost: in holes, wooden boxes, wire wool, plastic baskets or on the floor. Place several alternate layers of organic material (waste) and earth of equal thickness in the container. Always cover the earth, grass or leaves and damp them. You may add a small quantity of soil, ash or lime to the earth to stabilize it. Turn it to accelerate the process, if an odor is given off turn it over more frequently. Humidity must be between 50 and 60 % during the compost process. During the first few days, keep the temperature between 50° and 55°C, and between 55 and 60°C the following days, until the compost process has been completed. Heat should increase in two weeks, due to lack of nitrogen. Cut leaves do not contain nitrogen but they do contain manure, urea and ammonia sulfate. Design your compost container in accordance with minimum environmental hygiene requirements: two square meters for by one meter of height. Do not use meat, dairy products, etc for making compost as they attract rodents.

## ORGANIC GARBAGE---- COMPOST ---- HUMUS ---- VEGETABLE GARDENS.

Planetary Bio-Conscience.

"People are changing the resources in wastes faster than nature can turn them into resources again."

"Mankind can transform its conscience and evolve to a point that the energy of the system is reorganized. Life in PLANET EARTH."

"There is a very interesting theory that sees Earth as a living organism with its life cycles and its own defense mechanisms. Earth is much older than mankind, therefore wiser."

"If mankind becomes a virus, the defense mechanisms of this living organism that we call Earth, will be paralyzed without defending the integrity of the life system. Aren't tsunamis, melting of glaciers, flooding, earthquakes a form of bacteria?. The Planetary Bio-conscience impels the consensus and the mutual understanding of all the peoples of the world; that all being things are happy and there be peace on Earth, for a planet's eco-village." From: Om Vivere Argentina.

# BIBLIOGRAPHY

Guire, Georges, Dr., Alimentación y dietética.

Diamond Harvey y Marilyn, Anti-dieta. Editorial Urano

Chavez. M., Margarita. Nutrición Efectiva=A comida vegetariana.

Rius, El Cocinero Vegetariano, Editorial Grijalva.

Vda. De Culveaux, Ma., Alonso. México y su cocina Dietético Vegetariana.

Martín, Pol, La cocina fácil de Hoy, Editorial Brimar.

¿Qué cocinar?, Com. Nuniplex marqueting, Inc., Québec Farmer's group Canada.

Enciclopedia Salvat de la cocina. Salvat Editores, Pamplona, España.

Rouet Marcel. La salud por la comida. Editorial mensajero, España 1974

Doria Irma. La cocina macrobiótica. Editorial De Vichi. S.A., Barcelona, 1978

López Cortéz getuls Encarnación y G. Jordán getuls Ma. Luisa, El cocineno Vegetariano.

Gran Recetario Natura, Editorial Posada.

Jensen, Dr. Bernard, Manual Naturista. Editorial Yug.

Michán Shaya Manual Naturista. 1ª. Edición

Walker, Dr. Norman, Colon Health, Norwalk Press.

Walker, Dr. Norman W. Fresh Vegetables and Fruit juices, Norwalk Press.

Ganong, William F. Manual de Fisiología Médica, 4a. Edición Editorial el Manual Moderno 1974

Alonso, Dr. Eduardo. 50 lecciones de Medicina Natural. Editorial Kier, Argentina.

Pérez Rafael Lazaeta. Manual de alimentación sana. 2ª. Edición, Ediciones Lazaeta.

Scala, Dr. James. Como alcanzar la longevidad, Best Seller, Editorial Lasser Press-Mexicana S.A. de C.V.

Deal, Dr. Sheldon. New life through Nutrition.

Cot, Dr. Allan. Ayuno: la dieta máxima, 1ª. Edición, Editorial Diana, 1977

Consejero Médico familiar, Reader's Digest.

Brevet Rueff, Claudine. Las Medicinas Sagradas, Editorial Argos, S.A. Barcelona, España.

Vander, Dr. Adrian. Plantas Medicinales, Editorial Adrian Vander Peel, 1982.

Pérez, Ma. Del Socorro. Folleto: Hábitos de vida, hábitos de muerte.

Villacís, R. Dr. Luís. Plantas medicinales de México, Editorial Epoca, S.A. 1ª. Edición.

Martínez, Máximo, Plantas Mexicanas, 1ª Edición Editorial Fondo de Cultura Económica 1987

García, M. G. Manual de Botánica Medicinal.

Nahmias Francoise, La miel cura y sana, Editorial De Vecchi, S.A. Barcelona 1980

Jensen, Dr. Bernard. Semillas y Germinados, Editorial Yug.

Moore Lappe Frances, La Dieta Ecológica, Ballantine Books.

Rius, El yerberito ilustrado, Biblioteca Natura, 11ª. Edición Editorial Posada.

Propiedades curativas de los alimentos, Biblioteca Natura, Editorial Posada.

Alimentación integral para una vida sana, Biblioteca Natura, Editorial Posada 1978.

Revista Natura, varios números.

Deffes Caso Armando, Basura es la solución.

Caplan R, Our Herat, ourselves.

# About the Author

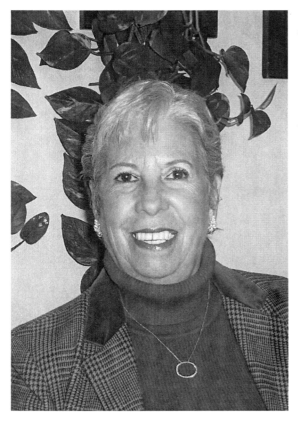

Julia Maitret was born in San Rafael, Veracruz, Mexico. She made her studies in Puebla, Mexico, until she obtained her Accountant degree. She then got an academic degree in Psicology and another in Interior Design. After a while she decided to go back to the University to pursue her degree in Humanities which she wasn't able to obtain due to the loss of two of her children; her oldest son at the age of 19 and her youngest at the age of 4.

She's convinced that her change to vegetarianism gave her the strength to endure and overcome her pain. Her husband and her, as a couple, couldn't overcome it together and got a divorce.

She's been a vegetarian for 34 years and has been studying about nutrition for over 40 years.

Printed in the United States
144523LV00001B/8/P